Tell Me What to Eat
If I Have
Acid Reflux

Tell Me What to Eat
If I Have
Acid Reflux

Revised Edition

Nutrition You Can Live With

By Elaine Magee, MPH, RD

Foreword by Anthony A. Starpoli, MD

 New Page Books
A Division of The Career Press, Inc.
Franklin Lakes, NJ

TELL ME WHAT TO EAT IF I HAVE ACID REFLUX
EDITED AND TYPESET BY GINA TALUCCI
CONTRIBUTOR: ANTHONY STARPOLI, MD
Cover design by Lu Rossman/Digi Dog Design NYC
Printed in the U.S.A. by Book-mart Press

To order this title, please call toll-free 1-800-CAREER-1 (NJ and Canada: 201-848-0310) to order using VISA or MasterCard, or for further information on books from Career Press.

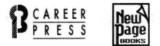

The Career Press, Inc., 3 Tice Road, PO Box 687,
Franklin Lakes, NJ 07417
www.careerpress.com
www.newpagebooks.com

Library of Congress Cataloging-in-Publication Data

Magee, Elaine.
    Tell me what to eat if I have acid reflux : nutrition you can live with / by Elaine Magee. —Rev. ed.
        p. cm.
    Includes index.
    ISBN 978-1-60163-019-3
        1. Gastroesophageal reflux—Popular works. 2. Gastroesophageal reflux—Diet therapy. I. Title.

RC815.7.M34 2008
616.3' 240654--dc22

                                                        2008021181

Contents

Foreword

Worldwide, 18 percent of people experience gastroesophageal reflux disease, also known as GERD, and commonly known as acid reflux. The most common symptom of reflux is heartburn, and it affects 7 to 10 percent of the U.S. population on a daily basis. Although medical science has made significant advances in the treatment of gastroesophageal reflux disease (GERD), it remains a chronic and relapsing condition.

The fact is that GERD is often undiagnosed and unrecognized. Compared to the multitude afflicted, a small number seek medical advice. Self-medication is common, and temporary relief of symptoms can be misleading. Complications to GERD can be masked by asymptomatic (a decrease in symptoms) response. It is well known that those patients with long-standing reflux may actually have fewer symptoms with time, yet the disease process may progress unbeknownst to the patient. The importance of making a specific diagnosis of GERD cannot be overemphasized.

Since the first edition of this book, the wide spectrum of reflux disease has been better exposed. The term *acid reflux* is used synonymously with GERD. More recent research data suggests that GERD is composed of nonacid reflux, as well as acid reflux.

Awareness of nonacid reflux emerged from GERD patients taking acid-lowering medications who continued to have symptoms despite their drug therapy. When evaluated it was found that these patients can still experience reflux symptoms that are of a nonacid nature, despite medical therapy. Nonacid reflux in this scenario can occur in 35 to 45 percent of patients who do not fully respond to drug therapy for reflux.

GERD continues to affect quality of life, and the bidirectional relationship between sleep and reflux is most interesting. Patients with poor sleep patterns can worsen their reflux, and those with poorly controlled GERD can have a disturbed sleep pattern.

A growing body of research data continues to point to GERD as a major risk factor for the development of cancer of the esophagus. The incidence of esophageal cancer has grown exponentially since the 1970s, which makes patients with the mildest forms of reflux desire to know more about their disease. Although medical and surgical therapies are widely available, reflux patients desire to play an active role in their care and make a quest to learn more about the disease and what they can do for themselves.

Most practitioners, like me, are short-handed with regard to providing patients with detailed dietary and lifestyle advice. I am impressed with patients' desire to understand the process behind their affliction. Most physicians are not well equipped to offer patients new approaches to diet and lifestyle. It is those things that are cornerstones to the successful management of any medical problem, including acid reflux. Proper nutrition can help combat the obesity that has been identified as an independent risk factor for developing GERD.

Tell Me What to Eat If I Have Acid Reflux offers a comprehensive review of the mechanisms behind reflux disease and explores its many manifestations. This review edition covers the medical and procedural aspects of GERD therapy, and provides an update on the newer nonsurgical procedures for GERD as well.

Most importantly, Elaine Magee's presentation of acid reflux disorders provides the reader with an easy understanding of reflux disorders and provides a patient oriented, realistic strategy to controlling the condition. Her writing offers the reader a sense that they can be in control, and provides a healthy direction for any person struggling with acid reflux.

Once again, Elaine Magee has thoroughly researched the nutrition basis for the treatment of acid reflux disease and gives practical guidelines that will lead patients to a better quality of life. I recommend this book to all my reflux patients as the perfect adjunct to their care.

Anthony A. Starpoli, MD
director of Gastroesophageal Reflux and Endosurgery
St. Vincents Catholic Medical Center-Manhattan
Attending, Gastroenterology
Lenox Hill Hospital New York, New York

Introduction

Heartburn isn't just a small inconvenience; it is very painful and can keep you from quality sleep and from doing your work. But then if you are one of the 60 million Americans who get heartburn at least once a month, you probably already knew this.

Heartburn happens when the lining of the esophagus comes in contact with too much stomach juice (contains stomach acid), which can produce a burning pain and injure the esophagus. There is a valve that connects the end of the esophagus with the beginning of the stomach, which normally functions to keep the stomach acid where it belongs—in the stomach. But in people with frequent heartburn, this valve, the lower esophageal sphincter muscle (LES), relaxes too frequently, allowing the stomach acid to splash up into the esophagus.

But you don't have to take this lying down, literally! There are foods you can choose and foods you can lose to help head off heartburn. A recent national survey conducted by the National Heartburn Alliance (NHBA), revealed that 92 percent of frequent heartburn sufferers point to food as the primary cause of their digestive discomfort. "The good news for sufferers is that anecdotal evidence indicates that changing your diet can significantly decrease the number of heartburn episodes," states the NHBA.

Enter acid reflux—when heartburn becomes an occasional or frequent visitor.

All you have to do is say the words *heartburn* or *acid reflux* and suddenly everyone with whom you speak either has it or knows several people who do. I think I've hit the magical age of acid reflux, because now that I am 40, I hear more and more about people being diagnosed with it. Do I personally suffer from it? Not yet, but I do know plenty of good friends and family members who have been suffering from it. That's why I made sure to include a book on acid reflux in my Tell Me What to Eat medical nutrition series.

Acid reflux is a disease that should not be ignored or self-treated. But what concerns me is that nearly half of acid reflux sufferers do not know that what they have been experiencing is an actual disease.

In studies that measure emotional well-being, people with unresolved acid reflux often report worse scores than people with other chronic diseases such as diabetes, high blood pressure, peptic ulcer, or angina.

Here's the good news: Acid reflux is generally a treatable disease. Now, here's even better news: Most people with acid reflux have a mild form of the disease that can be controlled through lifestyle changes and medication.

If you think you may have acid reflux and you haven't already consulted a physician about it, that's the first step you need to take. The second step is working with your doctor to put together the best available treatment plan for you. No matter what medical course of action you and your doctor decide to take, the diet and lifestyle tips in this book will be a nice compliment.

Don't suffer needlessly. Find out for sure if you have acid re-flux, then get the help that you need to feel great again. Reading this book will certainly help put you on the right track—the heartburn-free track!

Publisher's Note

This book is not intended as a substitute for medical advice. Readers are encouraged to consult with a doctor before following this or any other dietary advice.

Chapter 1

Everything You Ever Wanted to Ask Your Doctor About Acid Reflux

True, the majority of the book is devoted to the lifestyle and diet treatment options for acid reflux. Don't worry, we'll get to that. *Acid reflux* is the best-known term for gastroesophageal reflux disease, otherwise known as GERD. For our discussion we will use the term *acid reflux*, but know that reflux can be made up of acid and nonacid reflux. But first, you need to understand the who, what, where, why, and how of acid reflux. What is acid reflux? How do I got *relief* from my symptoms? What are my medical options—from over-the-counter products to surgery—and what are their side effects and risks? Answering these questions is what this chapter is all about. It's about everything you ever wanted to ask your doctor about acid reflux—if you could ever have his or her undivided attention for about an hour or two.

Q: Who has acid reflux?

If you have acid reflux, you are definitely not alone. More than 15 million Americans suffer from heartburn daily (a major symptom of acid reflux), with an additional 45 million having heartburn at least once a month. Do the math. That quickly adds up to at least 10 percent of Americans having some degree of acid reflux disease.

Q: What's going on inside my body with acid reflux?

When you have acid reflux, acid from the stomach flows backward up into the esophagus. So the word *acid* comes from the stomach acid, and the word *reflux* comes from the "backward flow" (or refluxing) of this stomach acid into the lower esophagus. Sounds rather simple doesn't it? But this little backsplash of the stomach acid contents comprised of acid and nonacidic material can injure the lining of your esophagus and wreak havoc in your life. It can disturb sleep, make you very uncomfortable after meals, cause a great deal of pain and discomfort, and, when untreated, can lead to serious complications.

When the body is functioning normally, this backsplash of stomach acid should never even reach as far up as the esophagus. You see, our bodies have a muscular valve called the lower esophageal sphincter, which connects the lower end of the esophagus with the upper end of the stomach. Food is only supposed to flow downward from the esophagus into the stomach where the food proceeds to get digested. But with acid reflux disease, this valve relaxes too frequently and allows some stomach acid to flow backward up into the esophagus.

Q: Is there a cure for acid reflux?

Acid reflux is a recurrent and chronic disease that does not resolve itself and go away. Anyone who has suffered from it for many years can tell you that. But long-term medical and lifestyle therapy is usually effective; it helps relieve symptoms in most people. Treatment options include lifestyle changes, medications, surgery, or a combination of those options—most help to keep the stomach acid from entering the lower esophagus.

Q: What is the most common symptom?

Heartburn! Thirty to 45 minutes after a heavy meal, heartburn hits. When excessive amounts of acid reflux enter the lower esophagus, the biggest result is heartburn, which is described as a feeling of burning discomfort right behind the breastbone (or heart) area of the body, that moves up toward the neck and throat. The burning can last for several hours and is often the worst after meals. Having heartburn every now and then isn't necessarily acid reflux or a health "problem." But when heartburn is frequent (two or more times a week) or accompanied by other symptoms (food sticking in the throat, blood loss, or weight loss), that's when acid reflux becomes the diagnosis. Some people even taste the sour stomach acid in the back of the throat.

Q: What are the other symptoms of acid reflux?

Besides heartburn, other common symptoms of acid reflux can include:

- a sensation of food coming back into the mouth accompanied by an acidic or sour taste.
- hoarseness.
- chronic cough.
- chronic asthma.
- belching.
- bloating.

Q: What can I do for just occasional heartburn?

For occasional heartburn, many people have found relief by using over-the-counter medicines and making some changes in their food habits and lifestyle, which include:

- avoiding foods and beverages that may be contributing to heartburn (more on this in Chapter 2).
- quitting smoking.
- trimming off some extra pounds if you are overweight. (I know from personal experience—this is absolutely "easier said than done.") This is so important that Chapter 4 is entirely devoted to it.
- eating your last meal or snack three hours or more before you go to sleep. When you allot that much time, there is a better chance that you are going to sleep on a somewhat empty stomach. The contents of the stomach should be small, and therefore less likely to splash up into the esophagus when you lay down.

Q: Is heartburn just the result of bad habits or does it have a physical cause?

You may be able to point your finger at bad eating habits for "occasional" heartburn. Habits such as overeating during meals that are high in fat, over-indulging in alcohol, and eating certain irritating food products such as citrus juices, spicy tomato products, or chocolates, can cause heartburn—even in healthy individuals. But when you have more frequent heartburn and other symptoms of acid reflux, there is more likely a physical cause.

Q: What about pregnant women and heartburn?

For many women, their first introduction to heartburn is their last few months of pregnancy, but there is a good explanation for this. The growing baby presses on the stomach, which can cause backward flow of stomach contents into the esophagus. The bad news is this type of heartburn is often resistant to dietary changes and even antacids. The good news is, once the baby is born, the heartburn most often disappears.

Q: What is the key to relieving the symptoms?

If the physical cause of acid reflux is the stomach acid refluxing into the esophagus from the stomach, then suppressing that acid and keeping it from irritating esophageal tissue is the key in relieving the symptoms and letting the irritated tissue heal.

Q: When are symptoms the worst?

Esophageal acid exposure in people with esophagitis is typically more frequent during the day than at night, and especially after meals. Irritation and injury of esophageal tissue can take place directly after meals, because that's when acid is released from the stomach and the esophageal sphincter can have a tendency to relax, allowing the stomach acid to splash into the esophagus.

For others, heartburn tends to rear its ugly head at bedtime. That's when all the foods and beverages we probably shouldn't have had in excess come back and haunt us. When you lie down to go to sleep, you shift the stomach from an up-and-down position to a sideways position, and suddenly the opening to the esophagus is level with the rest of the stomach and its contents.

Q: What are my treatment options?

Acid reflux is usually treated with a combination of diet and lifestyle changes, over-the-counter or prescription medications, and in some cases, surgery. Most doctors start with the least invasive, least expensive options, such as over-the-counter medicines and changing some troublesome lifestyle habits, and then work their way to more intensive treatments, such as prescription medications and surgery.

Q: How is heartburn different from GERD/acid reflux?

Everyone experiences heartburn sometime in his or her life. But when the heartburn progresses from occasional heartburn to more than twice a week heartburn…or the heartburn is associated with any of the various complications (such as food sticking, weight loss, low blood count), your heartburn has most likely developed into acid reflux disease.

Q: Which drugs are best for acid reflux and how do they work?

The following drugs offer effective treatment to "some" or "most" people. However, keep in mind that none of the current drugs used to treat acid reflux actually cures it. They help control symptoms and some also allow the esophagus to heal if there is tissue damage. Even when the drugs relieve symptoms completely, the condition usually reoccurs within months after the drugs are discontinued.

Q: What do over-the-counter antacids and foaming agents (alginic acid) do?

Antacids are great for rapidly relieving heartburn symptoms. They work directly in the stomach to decrease the acidity of the reflux liquid irritating the esophagus. They also help neutralize the area inside the esophagus. When antacids and a foaming agent are combined, they produce a foam barrier in the stomach, which floats over the contents of the stomach, preventing acid from splashing up into the esophagus. They do not heal esophagitis or prevent complications of acid reflux.

Q: What are the side effects of long-term use of antacids?

- Diarrhea from some antacids (Milk of Magnesia) and constipation from others (Amphogel, Alternagel). Aluminum and magnesium salts are used together in Mylanta and Maalox to help balance the side effects of diarrhea and constipation.

- Constipation can be caused by calcium carbonate (Tums, Titralac, and Alka-2). These over-the-counter antacids are a source of calcium, and in rare cases, can lead to too much calcium in the blood, leading to kidney failure.

- A change in the way the body breaks down and uses calcium.

- An increased risk of kidney stones.

- A buildup of magnesium in the body can be serious for patients with kidney disease.

If antacids are needed for more than three weeks, a doctor should be consulted.

Q: Can they interact with other drugs I might be taking?

Antacids can reduce the absorption of certain drugs (tetracycline, ciprofloxacin (Cipro), propanolol (Inderal), captopril (Capoten), and H2 blockers), so please let your doctor know if you are using antacids (even if you only use them every now and then). It will help to take the other drugs one hour before or three hours after you take the antacid.

Q: H2 blockers—what do they do?

H2 blockers (also called H2 receptor antagonists), help inhibit acid secretion in the stomach (which helps reduce the stomach acid that tends to worsen symptoms). Specifically, they work to block the type II histamine receptor that is one of the mechanisms controlling acid production. They work in about 30 minutes and last up to eight hours.

There are over-the-counter H2 blockers and prescription H2 blockers. The over-the-counter version does not relieve symptoms as quickly as antacids, but they last longer. In other words, they may be slow to start, but once they get going, they help your acid reflux for a long time.

H2 blockers have been the traditional drug treatment in acid reflux because many of them can be an effective short-term therapy for resistant acid reflux symptoms. In most studies on H2 blockers, where the participants were taking these drugs twice a day, symptoms were eliminated in up to half of the people. In one particular study (participants took ranitidine, 150 mg, twice a day), people were healed of their esophagitis within six weeks.

When taking these drugs keep three things in mind:

1. High doses are more effective than the more standard doses.

2. Taking them twice a day is more effective than taking them once a day.

3. H2 blockers are generally less expensive than proton pump inhibitors (see page 28 to find out more about proton pump inhibitors).

Over-the-counter version

A lower-dose, over-the-counter version of H2 blockers is available to help control "episodes" of heartburn, under the names cimetidine (100 mg), famotidine (10 mg), nizatidine (75 mg), and ranitidine (75 mg). They take longer to act than antacids (symptom relief may take 30 to 60 minutes), but they last longer.

You've probably seen these advertised on TV

Commercials abound for a couple of the drugs in this category. You know them by name—Tagamet HB, Pepcid AC, and Zantac 75.

For Tagamet (cimetidine), the prescribed dose is usually 300 mg, three times a day for four to six weeks, and many people experience improvement after two to four weeks. Because antacids reduce the absorption of Tagamet, make sure you take your antacids an hour before or after Tagamet is taken. Some take the H2 blocker before eating and antacids after eating.

For Zantac (ranitidine HCl), the prescribed dose is usually 150 mg two times a day for four to six weeks depending on the response. For people whose symptoms mainly appear at night, a single dose of 300 mg taken at bedtime might do the trick.

Warning: Even though these drugs are available without a prescription from your doctor, you should seek medical attention for persistent heartburn.

Side effects

These drugs, for the most part, have few side effects. Headache is the most common one cited. Other side effects reported are mild, temporary diarrhea, dizziness, and a rash; liver and nerve disease exacerbate these side effects. Another concern is that long-term acid suppression with these drugs may cause cancerous changes in the stomach in people who also have untreated *H. pylori* infections (this also goes for long-term use of proton pump inhibitor drugs).

- Tagamet (cimetidine) interacts with a number of common medications (phenytoin, theophylline, and wafarin). Long-term use of excessive doses (more than 3 g a day) of cimetidine may cause impotence or breast enlargement (these problems reverse after the drug is discontinued).
- Zantac (ranitidine) interferes with very few drugs.
- Axid (famotidine and nizatidine), the latest H2 blocker, is nearly free of side effects or drug interactions.

Promotility agents

These drugs are used for mild to moderate acid reflux symptoms and they are especially good at decreasing heartburn symptoms at night. They are often paired with H2 blockers to work together—they act in different ways to reduce symptoms. Although prescription H2 blockers moderately suppress acid, promotility agents:

- increase the strength of the lower esophageal sphincter muscle.

- speed up emptying of the stomach contents and enhance esophageal motility or movement through the esophagus. (Cisapride, bethanechol, erythromycin, and metoclopramide are the four promotility agents currently available.)

Side effects

Erythromycin is an antibiotic and can cause nausea and diarrhea.

Metoclopramide can include side effects such as drowsiness, anxiety, agitation, and motor restlessness in up to 30 percent of patients. The effect of this drug is more pronounced when given intravenously rather than orally.

Cisapride (Propulsid) should be avoided by people with certain disorders including, but not limited to, almost any heart disease, kidney failure, apnea, emphysema, chronic bronchitis, advanced cancer, and conditions that increase the risk for electrolyte disorders (imbalances in potassium, magnesium, sodium, or calcium). And it should be used with caution in people with liver disorders. The Food and Drug Administration states that Propulsid should not be used by people taking antiallergy, antiangina, and antiarrhythmics (irregular heart rhythm drugs) medicines, or antibiotics, antidepressants, antifungals, antinausea, antipsychotics, or protease inhibitors (for HIV). The FDA also advises that Propulsid should not be prescribed to anyone with a history of irregular heartbeats, abnormal electrocardiogram, heart disease, kidney disease, lung disease, eating disorder, dehydration, persistent vomiting, or low levels of potassium, calcium, or magnesium.

Proton pump inhibitors

Proton pump inhibitors claim that they heal erosive esophagitis more rapidly than H2 blockers. They do this by decreasing the acidity of the stomach contents by inhibiting an enzyme necessary for acid secretion.

Doctors are now using these as the mainstay for acid reflux treatment, because they provide potent acid suppression—a better way to help relieve symptoms and to let irritated tissues get a chance to heal more completely. These drugs may help control meal-stimulated acid secretion, but acid reflux during sleep can still occur with patients who are taking these drugs.

The proton pump inhibitor drugs available by prescription include omeprazole (Prilosec), esoemprazole (Nexium), lansoprazole (Prevacid), rabeprazole (Aciphex), pantoprazole (Protonix), and Zegerid (a newer combination of omeprazole and sodium bicarbonate). For the most part, they work similarly, and they are only used when symptoms are severe or when there is damage to the esophagus lining.

What they do

These drugs maintain a stomach acid level pH of more than 4.0. They do this by almost completely turning off the acid producing pumps of the stomach. In the right doses, proton pump inhibitor medications are the most effective agents for healing esophagitis and preventing complications (something the other drugs aren't as good at doing). They also provide a more complete rapid relief of acid reflux symptoms. With the exception of rabeprazole, which will have an onset of action in about 40 minutes, drugs of this class will take about two to six hours to begin having an effect of lowering acid production. After 24 hours they will have a more profound acid-lowering effect than any other class.

Some studies have shown that the use of lansoprazole and drugs such as omeprazole (two proton pump inhibitor drugs currently available in the United States) leads to symptom relief in a majority of patients and healing of the esophagus in roughly more than 80 percent of the participants (*Gastroenterology*, 1997).

Recent studies show erosive esophagitis healing rates were positively related to better stomach acid suppression, and this control correlated with lower final daytime and nighttime heartburn and acid regurgitation symptom scores.

What they don't do

They may have little or no effect on regurgitation or controlling asthmatic symptoms. In other words they do not control the mechanical aspect of reflux

Are they safe?

Reported side effects of the drug omeprazole and similar drugs of this class, although uncommon, are headache, diarrhea, abdominal pain, and nausea. Certain medications, whose absorption into the body depends on a certain stomach acid level, may not work as well when taking proton pump inhibitors as well as the promotility agents. They should not be used unless necessary by pregnant women or nursing mothers, and they appear to be safe for children with severe acid reflux.

Q: When should I discuss my heartburn with my doctor?

Heartburn is one of those medical issues where people tend to treat themselves with over-the-counter medicine and then go into a "wait and see" mode—they wait and see if it comes back or gets worse. It's always best to check in with a doctor and let them know what you are experiencing and what you have been using to treat it. If you have heartburn several times a week, it is often a sign of acid reflux or GERD. You should see a doctor or gastroenterologist if you have heartburn on a weekly basis, but the following are what I call "sounding the alarm" acid reflux symptoms, which are definitely signs that you should see a doctor asap:

- Difficulty swallowing or a sharp pain with swallowing.
- Heartburn symptoms starting at a later age (age 50-plus).
- Vomiting.
- Blood in your stool.
- Unexplained weight loss or loss of appetite.
- Having a history of iron deficiency anemia.

Q: Could other medicines you are taking be making your acid reflux worse?

Medications you might be taking for other health problems can actually aggravate your acid reflux.

Check with your doctor to make sure you aren't taking the type of prescriptions that could be making your acid reflux worse.

Some cause the lower esophageal sphincter to relax. These are:

- calcium channel blockers.
- anti-cholinergics.
- alpha-adrenergic agonists.
- dopamine.
- sedatives.
- common pain relievers.

Some can weaken the peristaltic action of the esophagus and can slow stomach emptying. These are:

- calcium channel blockers.
- anti-cholinergics.

Some can cause damage to the esophagus lining, such as:

- Alendronate (Fosamax, an anti-osteoporosis drug). Take this drug with 6 to 8 ounces of water (not juice, carbonated water, or mineral water) on an empty stomach in the morning and remain upright for 30 minutes afterward.
- Potassium and iron pills can be corrosive and cause ulcers in the esophagus.
- Antibiotics can make the mucus membrane more vulnerable to acids.

Non-steroidal anti-inflammatory drugs (NSAID) are known for potentially causing ulcers in the stomach. But can they also harm the esophagus? One recent study found that elderly people who took these drugs and had acid reflux were at higher risk for acid reflux complications (particularly strictures, abnormal narrowing of the esophagus, and Barrett's esophagus).

If you have been taking non-steroidal anti-inflammatory drugs, you might be twice as likely to develop acid reflux disease, according to presenters at the annual meeting of the American College of Rheumatology. The results are from a study focused on people taking prescription NSAIDs for osteoarthritis. These drugs may contribute to acid reflux by relaxing the lower esophageal sphincter muscle, allowing the stomach contents to more easily find their way into the esophagus (*RN*, March 2000; vol. 63 i3: 96).

There are dozens of non-steroidal anti-inflammatory drugs, some of which are going to look very familiar.

- Aspirin.
- Ibuprofen (Motrin, Advil, Nuprin, Rufen).
- Naproxen (Aleve).

- Piroxicam (Feldene).
- Diflunisal (Dolobid).
- Indomethacin (Indocin).
- Flurbiprofen (Ansaid).
- Ketorolac (Toradol).
- Ketoprofen (Acron, Orudis KT).
- Diclofenac (Voltaren).

Note: If you have acid reflux, taking an "occasional" aspirin or other nonsteroidal anti-inflammatory drug will probably not harm you. But if you want to avoid them, Tylenol (acetaminophen) is a good alternative.

Q: Is that an aspirin in your throat?

Sometimes acid reflux symptoms can appear simply because pills containing irritating chemicals become trapped in the esophagus and eventually dissolve. It can also happen with vitamin C supplements and antibiotics such as tetracycline.

Q: Which tests are used to evaluate acid reflux?

If your symptoms don't improve with prescription medications, your doctor may use one or more of the following tests to gather more information. An acid reflux exam often includes an endoscopy (described in the following). It takes about 15 to 30 minutes for the procedure.

Upper GI Series

You are asked to swallow a liquid barium mixture and the radiologist uses a fluoroscope to watch the barium as it travels down your esophagus and into the stomach. X rays are usually taken as needed. This test provides limited information about possible acid reflux, but helps rule out other possible diagnoses, such as peptic ulcers and plays a minor role in the evaluation of acid reflux. It may be helpful in the evaluation of swallowing disorders.

Endoscopy

After you have been sedated, a small, lighted, flexible tube is passed through the mouth, and into the esophagus and stomach to look for abnormalities like inflammation or irritation of the lining of the esophagus. This is thought to be the best way to identify esophagitis, Barrett's esophagus, and all inflammation of the esophagus. If the endoscopy finds anything suspicious, a small sample of the esophagus lining is often taken for further testing (biopsy). Newer forms of endoscopy use a technique called narrow band imaging (NBI) in combination with high definition (HD) that allows for a very accurate imaging of the lining of the esophagus and stomach and, if necessary, helps target suspicious areas of the esophagus and stomach for closer inspection and possible biopsy.

Esophageal Maonometry or Esophageal pHreflux testing

A small flexible tube is passed through the nose into the esophagus and stomach to measure pressures and function of the esophagus (manometry). Twenty-four hour reflux testing that measures the degree of acid that refluxes into the esophagus can also be performed. The newest technology utilizes both pH and impedance sensors that allows the detection of acid and nonacid reflux. It is the nonacid reflux that is mostly responsible for the patients that continue to suffer reflux despite medical therapy with acid lowering drugs.

When anti-reflux surgery is suggested

If medical treatment fails, surgery may be in order, especially for young patients who want to avoid decades of taking stomach medications. Currently, anti-reflux surgery is performed using the laparoscopic fundoplication, where the upper part of the stomach is wrapped around the esophagus to increase the pressure on the esophageal sphincter and keep acid in the stomach. This procedure has a 10-year success rate of about 80 to 90 percent. People with an impaired lower esophageal sphincter (the valve connecting the lower esophagus to the upper stomach) are most likely to benefit from surgery.

Side effects (usually temporary) or complications associated with surgery occur in 5 to 20 percent of patients (International Foundation for Functional Gastrointestinal Disorders), the most common being difficulty swallowing, the inability to burp or vomit, and the gas-belch-bloat syndrome. Following this surgery, a small percentage of patients can also have an alteration in their bowel habits with a tendency toward diarrhea.

Anti-reflux surgery may not fix the problem forever, either. It can break down, similar to hernia repairs in the body. The recurrence rate is thought to be in the range of 10 to 30 percent throughout 20 years. In some people, even after surgery, their reflux symptoms persist to the point of needing to continue their medications anyway. Prior to any antireflux procedure, you must have a thorough evaluation that includes 24-hour reflux testing and esophageal motility testing.

New high-tech options

Since the year 2000, the world of gastrointestinal medicine and endoscopic (camera tube) technology has seen a variety of nonsurgical, endoscopic, and incisionless techniques that have been met with mixed reviews by the medical community.

At this time, there are two FDA approved devices that have clinical data to support their application in the treatment of reflux disease. These companies are C.R. Bard-Davol who developed and distribute the EndoCinch Suturing System that allows for stitches to be placed at the level of the lower sphincter valve between the stomach and the esophagus; the stitches create a set of pleats that tighten the valve.

NDO Surgical Inc. has developed a system called the Plicator. The device places two deep sutures that pass through the entire wall of the upper stomach right below the lower sphincter. This array of sutures creates a deep plication that most closely resembles the formal surgical procedure known as the Nissen fundoplication. Sham-controlled studies show the Plicator to be superior to the other nonsurgical approaches with more than two thirds of patients responding with fewer symptoms and reduction or elimination of medication. Although not as effective as surgery, the endoscopic approaches to reflux management can help properly selected patients who either do not completely respond to medical therapy, do not wish to take life-long drug therapy, experience side effects from acid lowering drugs, or have certain features of GERD that may benefit from strengthening of the lower sphincter valve. General anesthesia is usually not needed, and, although not risk free, carries lower risks than the more invasive anti-reflux surgery. Failure of a nonsurgical approach does not preclude having formal reflux surgery.

These procedures are performed on an outpatient basis and most return to work the next day.

Q: What are the complications of acid reflux?

Only about 20 percent of patients seen by primary care doctors have a complicated form of acid reflux disease, such as erosive esophagitis, peptic stricture, or Barrett's esophagus (a premalignant condition where there is a change in the membrane cells).

Even if you currently have milder symptoms of acid reflux, complications could be waiting for you down the road—especially if your acid reflux isn't being treated. Overall, about 20 percent of patients with acid reflux go on to develop complications such as:

- esophageal stricture (4 to 20 percent)—a narrowing or obstruction of the esophagus.
- ulceration (2 to 7 percent).
- hemorrhage or bleeding (more than 2 percent).
- Barrett's esophagus (10 to 15 percent)—a pre-cancer change in the lining of the esophagus. (*Patient Care*, 34 (2000): 26).

If you have the following symptoms, serious damage may have already occurred and immediate medical attention is required:

- Dysphasia: Difficulty swallowing or a feeling that food is trapped behind the breastbone. (Almost half of acid reflux patients report having trouble swallowing.)
- Bleeding: Vomiting blood or having tarry, black bowel movements (this may occur if ulcers have developed in the esophagus).
- Choking: The sensation of acid refluxed into the windpipe causing shortness of breath, coughing, or hoarseness of the voice.
- Weight loss.

Q: What is the most serious complication of chronic acid reflux?

Barrett's esophagus. The lining of the esophagus basically changes to resemble the lining of the intestine (due to chronic and constant exposure to stomach acid). This is actually the body's way of trying to protect the esophagus from acid by replacing its normal lining cells with cells similar to the intestinal lining. Although patients often say their heartburn has actually improved with Barrett's esophagus, it is a pre-cancerous condition carrying with it a 30-fold increased risk of developing esophageal cancer. A new study (*Gastroenterology*, 2007) discovered that excessive abdominal fat increases the risk of Barrett's esophagus by 2.4 times compared to people who were not as large around the middle. According to Dr. Thomas L. Vaughan with the Fred Hutchinson Cancer Research Center in Seattle, this partially explains why men (who tend to put excess body fat around the mid-section) experience such a higher risk of developing Barrett's esophagus and esophageal cancer than women.

Can acid reflux be making my asthma worse?

Yes it can. Some researchers estimate that about half of asthmatic patients also have acid reflux. How do you know if acid reflux is making your asthma worse? Here are some clues:

1. Did your asthma appear for the first time as an adult?
2. Does your asthma seem to get worse after meals, lying down, or exercise?
3. Does your asthma occur mainly at night?

If you answered yes to the three clues, here's some good news. Treatment of your acid reflux can make a difference in your asthma symptoms (it has in about 70 percent of patients). Some experts believe that the acid leaking from the lower esophagus stimulates the nerves running along the neck into the chest, causing bronchial constriction and difficulty breathing. It's also possible that a small amount of acid may be breathed in, consequently irritating the upper airway and triggering asthma symptoms.

What comes first, the chicken or the egg? It could be the other way around for some people. Could the asthma be giving you acid reflux? Experts are still figuring this out, but wonder whether the coughing and sneezing with asthmatic attacks can cause changes in the chest and trigger reflux. It is also possible that certain asthmatic drugs (taken to dilate the airways) may relax the lower esophageal sphincter and contribute to acid reflux.

If you are asthmatic and you don't think your stomach acid is refluxing into your esophagus, you may want to think again. Researcher Susan Harading, with the Sleep/Wake Disorders Center at the University of Alabama, found that 62 percent of the asthmatic patients they studied who *did not* have acid reflux symptoms, actually showed physical signs of stomach acid in the upper portion of their esophagus throughout a 24-hour period.

Exercise-induced asthma, by the way, does not appear to be related to acid reflux.

If you are asthmatic and have reflux symptoms, strongly consider reflux therapy. If you don't have symptoms, but your asthma is hard to control, talk to your physician about esophageal pH testing to determine if you are having some acid reflux without symptoms.

Q: What ear, nose, and throat problems could be linked to acid reflux?

Do you have:

- A chronic cough?
- Sore throat?
- Laryngitis with hoarseness? (This can happen when stomach acid reaches the larynx or voice box.)
- A tendency to clear your throat often?
- Growths on your vocal cords?

Acid reflux may be causing these problems. This entity under the GERD umbrella is referred to as laryngeal-pharyngeal reflux, or LPR. If these problems have not gotten better with standard treatments, ask you doctor whether they could be happening as a result of an underlying problem with acid reflux. The treatment of LPR with an acid-lowering drug has not been all that successful and requires lengthy periods of therapy.

Q: Can acid reflux relapse after the esophagus has healed?

Yes. Acid reflux tends to be chronic (of long duration) and relapsing. Eighty percent of people with healed esophagitis experience a relapse within eight weeks after the treatment has ended. And 75 percent of people who had negative endoscopy results after finishing successful short-term therapy with the medication omeprazole experience relapsing symptoms within six months. Those statistics will sober you up real quick. That's why preventing relapse is a top concern with acid reflux—it's right up there with relieving symptoms and healing esophagitis.

Q: What does hiatal hernia have to do with acid reflux?

Hiatal hernia is when the upper part of the stomach moves up into the chest through a small opening in the diaphragm (the muscle separating the stomach from the chest).

What can cause hiatal hernia? Coughing, vomiting, straining, or sudden physical exertion can all cause increased pressure in the abdomen area, which can result in hiatal hernia. Being obese or pregnant can make hiatal hernia more likely. Many otherwise-healthy people age 50-plus have a small hiatal hernia, but it can happen to people at any age.

Although hiatal hernias can impair the lower esophageal sphincter function, recent studies have failed to find that this directly causes acid reflux disease. Many people with hiatal hernia have neither reflux nor esophagitis. But the people who happen to have both acid reflux and hiatal hernia do tend to have the more severe acid reflux.

Q: Am I having chest pain from acid reflux or my heart?

The early symptoms of a heart attack can be mistaken as heartburn, which is pretty scary. It is extremely important to know whether acid reflux or a more serious heart condition, such as angina or a heart attack, is causing your chest pain. Both heart attacks and acid reflux can occur after a heavy meal has been eaten. You can even have both at the same time! Some patients with coronary artery disease may develop anginal chest pain from their acid reflux. Some experts believe that the acid in the esophagus of such patients may activate nerves that temporarily impair blood flow to the heart.

It's always best to have your chest pain checked out immediately by a physician, but here are some hints that can help you along the way. These are more likely to be associated with acid reflux:

- Pain that continues for hours.
- Pain behind the sturnum or breastbone without radiating to the side of your body.
- Pain that interrupts sleep, or is related to meals.
- Pain is relieved with antacid agents or H2 blockers.

Call 911 immediately if:

- You've never had heartburn before this, and your are experiencing chest pain and pressure.

- Antacids don't relieve the burning sensation in your chest within 10 to 15 minutes.

Along with what you think is heartburn, you are also experiencing:

- Shortness of breath.
- Sweating.
- Nausea.
- Dizziness.
- Fainting.
- General weakness.
- Pain radiating from your chest to your back, jaw, or arms.

These symptoms mean that you may be having a heart attack!

Q: How effective is lifestyle modification?

No matter how severe your acid reflux is, lifestyle modification is recommended, because it is a low cost and simple way to help improve symptoms and reduce the risk of relapse. In fact, 20 percent of people with mild to moderate acid reflux find that lifestyle changes improve their symptoms. But when people with acid reflux have esophagitis (inflammation of the esophagus), the most effective treatment is to reduce the acidity and the volume of potential reflux liquid by using acid-blocking medications.

Q: What types of lifestyle changes are we taking about?

If you smoke, ask yourself whether your smoking is contributing to your acid reflux symptoms.

If you drink alcohol, is it possible that your symptoms seem to get worse after you drink?

When you sleep, don't lie down for three hours after eating, which means if you normally go to sleep at 10 p.m., the dinner hour should be no later than 6 to 7 p.m. This basically decreases the amount of stomach contents and stomach acid available to reflux when you lie down. If you like to eat a snack at bedtime, don't. Anyone who snacks at bedtime is at high risk for acid reflux symptoms.

If you wear tight clothing, try not to. Tight clothing squeezes the stomach and pushes stomach acid up into the esophagus.

If you are overweight, try to trim down a little. Obesity could be contributing to your acid reflux because the extra weight being carried around your stomach can also put pressure on the stomach contents, which can push stomach acid up toward the esophagus.

When you eat, avoid foods that lower the tone of the esophagus valve (fats and chocolate) and foods that may irritate the damaged lining of the esophagus (citrus juice, tomato juice, and pepper). For more on food-related recommendations, see Chapter 2.

If you eat heavy meals, you are at risk for an attack of heartburn, particularly if you follow that heavy meal with a quick siesta by lying on your back (or bending over from the waist).

Q: How do I sleep with acid reflux?

For many people with acid reflux, nighttime is a living nightmare. A lot of this has to do with physically lying down, when suddenly the stomach content has easier access to the opening of the esophagus. There are several things you can do to make acid reflux heartburn less likely when you sleep:

- Go to bed no earlier than four hours after having eaten your last meal or snack.
- Elevate the head of your bed about 6 inches by placing blocks under the legs at the head of the bed or an under-mattress foam wedge (to raise the head about 6 to 10 inches). This slightly raises your esophagus

compared to your stomach, so the stomach contents aren't as likely to splash up against the opening to your esophagus when you are lying down.

• The "right" side is wrong! It helps to put your stomach in a better position when you sleep on your left side.

Doctors at Philadelphia's Graduate Hospital charted acid flow and sleep position in 10 people. Although sleeping on their backs led to frequent but brief attacks, sleeping on their right sides caused the most pain and damage, leaving the left side as the proper side to sleep on, because it caused the least acid flow of all. Although this study isn't the end all and be all, try to sleep on your left side.

Note: The most frequent symptoms of acid reflux are so common that they may not be associated with a disease. Self-diagnosis can lead to mistreatment. Consultation with a physician is essential to proper diagnosis and treatment of acid reflux.

The goals of acid reflux treatment are:

1. To bring the symptoms under control so you feel better.
2. To heal the esophagus of inflammation or injury.
3. To manage or prevent complications of acid reflux.
4. To keep acid reflux symptoms in remission, so that daily life is unaffected or minimally affected by the reflux.

Definitions

Esophagus: The esophagus is the 10-inch long tube linking the throat and the stomach.

Esophagitis: Mild to moderate irritation of the esophagus or an inflamed lining of the esophagus.

Q: How do I know if my heartburn is serious?

Three things measure the severity of heartburn:

1. How long does a given episode of heartburn last?
2. How often does my heartburn occur?
3. How intense is my heartburn when it occurs?

It will help to know the answers to these questions when you visit your doctor or gastroenterologist.

Clues that it may be something serious:

- Having heartburn at least twice a week.
- Heartburn doesn't get better with antacids or over-the-counter medicine.
- Heartburn is associated with food sticking, weight loss, or a low blood count.

Q: Why stop smoking?

If you smoke, tobacco is making your acid reflux worse. Tobacco does three things to encourage acid reflux:

1. Inhibits saliva—saliva helps coat and protect the esophagus.
2. Stimulates stomach acid production.
3. Relaxes the sphincter between the esophagus and the stomach, allowing stomach acid to splash up into the esophagus.

Q: How often are you reaching for over-the-counter relief?

If you are using an over-the-counter product more than twice a week, you should consult a doctor. The doctor can then confirm a specific diagnosis and develop a treatment plan with you, which might include the use of stronger prescription medicines, if necessary.

The severity of acid reflux depends on:

- Lower esophageal sphincter dysfunction.
- The type and amount of fluid brought up from the stomach into the esophagus.
- The neutralizing effect of saliva.

Q: What is GERD?

GERD stands for Gastro Esophageal Reflux Disease. It is more commonly known as acid reflux disease, but nonacid reflux plays a role as well.

Q: What is dyspepsia?

Up to half of acid reflux sufferers have dyspepsia—a medical term for "indigestion." Symptoms include heartburn, fullness in the stomach, and nausea after eating. These symptoms tend to increase during times of stress.

For your information

Certain medications can actually aggravate acid reflux symptoms. That's why it is vitally important to tell your doctor about any and all medications you are taking.

Q: Do liquid antacids work better than tablets?

It is generally believed that liquid antacids work faster and are more potent than tablets, but evidence suggests that they all work equally well.

Q: How do I know when my over-the-counter antacids or H2 blockers aren't enough?

Using over-the-counter antacids and H2 blockers to relieve heartburn, without seeing a doctor, may work well for occasional heartburn, but they should not be used daily. If they are, they could be hiding a more severe disease and complications of acid reflux. When used in excess, these products can get expensive and may have significant side effects.

If you have heartburn more than twice a week or heartburn associated with food sticking, weight loss, or low blood count—you need to see your doctor immediately.

When your symptoms improve, your condition could actually be worse!

Believe it or not, when the esophagus is damaged, heartburn symptoms actually tend to improve. That's why if you have ever suffered from persistent heartburn, you may still need to see a doctor.

Q: How can you prevent complications from acid reflux?

- Don't ignore persistent symptoms of heartburn and reflux.

- See your doctor early. The physical cause of acid reflux can then be treated, and the more serious complications of acid reflux can be avoided!

Q: Does having acid reflux increase your risk of cancer of the esophagus?

A recent study reported that people with acid reflux are at higher risk for a type of esophageal cancer (esophageal adenocarcinoma)—with or without developing Barrett's esophagus. A recent study (*New England Journal of Medicine*, 18 (1999): 825) found that people with a history of acid reflux had more than seven times the risk of esophageal adenocarcinoma, and people with long-standing or severe acid reflux had a 43 times greater risk. The overall incidence and associated mortality of esophageal cancer in the United States has increased 15 to 20 percent throughout the past three decades (Nat Clinical Gastro Hepato 4 (2006): 2–3).

Some experts suspect that bile (not stomach acid) refluxing into the esophagus may be increasing the risk for cancerous changes. Bile is a digestive fluid made up of water, bile salts, lecithin, and cholesterol that is normally stored in the gallbladder and released into the small intestine to help digest and absorb food components. There is an anti-reflux surgical procedure available that might be effective in suppressing both bile and acid reflux.

More about asthma

Asthma is a chronic disease affecting more than 17 million Americans. When you have an asthma attack, cells within your lungs overproduce mucus, clogging the airways. The bronchial tubes swell and the muscles surrounding them tighten, causing the airways to narrow, and making it very hard to breathe.

The simplest way to raise the head of your bed

BedBlox, a pair of specially designed plastic fixtures that are placed under the head of your bed, are now available online at *www.bedrisersales.com* for $39.95.

You can also make your own using a 4 × 4-inch piece of wood and nailing two jar caps the right distance apart to hold the legs or casters at the upper end of the bed. If you don't use jar caps, you risk being jolted from your slumber when the upper end of the bed rolls off the 4 × 4.

Chapter 2

Everything You Ever Wanted to Know About Food and Acid Reflux

You learn rather quickly by experience that when you eat or drink certain things in certain amounts, your acid reflux acts up. Wouldn't you like to know what those foods are right away, so you can be forewarned and perhaps forearmed (with medicines if need be)? The following chapter has everything you need to know about what you eat, how much you eat, and when you eat.

A little warning: Some of the food suggestions are going to be easier to swallow than others (literally). Experts agree people can respond differently to potential trigger food and drink—there are individual differences.

Q: What are the foods I need to be careful of now that I have acid reflux?

Fifteen years ago, the standard anti-reflux diet called for restricting foods that seemed to bring on or aggravate acid reflux symptoms—spicy foods, acidic foods, fatty foods, as well as coffee, tea, and cola drinks. Two extra foods were also on the list of food "no no's," because they were thought to lower the esophageal sphincter pressure, which would encourage stomach acid to reflux into the esophagus. What are those two foods? Get ready, because I can guarantee you aren't going to like this...peppermint and chocolate.

So is this 15-year-old anti-reflux diet still the gold standard? Yes, with some modifications. These are the foods/drinks that irritate acid reflux by either weakening the lower esophageal sphincter, increasing the acid content of the stomach, or bloating up the abdomen, causing pressure up toward the esophagus.

Foods that weaken the lower esophageal sphincter muscle encouraging acid reflux or heartburn, which should be eaten in smaller portions or limited:

- Fried or fatty foods.
- Coffee (including decaffeinated coffee, which increases acid content in the stomach).
- Caffeinated tea and cola drinks (increase acid content in the stomach).
- Alcoholic beverages. (Although some studies have shown that small amounts of alcohol may actually protect the mucosal layer.)
- Chocolate.
- Peppermint and spearmint.
- Garlic.
- Onions.

Foods that increase the acid content in the stomach, which should be limited or consumed in small portions:

- All caffeinated drinks (coffee, tea, and soda with caffeine).
- Coffee (including decaf coffee).

Food that can irritate a damaged esophageal lining and should be limited or eaten in small portions:

- Citrus fruits and juices.
- Tomato products.
- Chili peppers.
- Pepper.

Foods that can bloat up the abdomen causing pressures that force acid to back up into the esophagus:

- All carbonated beverages.

I know the previous list looks rather ominous. If you like Italian food, how can you get through a meal without a ton of garlic, onions, or tomato sauce? And if you are like most red-blooded Americans, how do you get through the morning without a cup of coffee? And what about alcohol? If you enjoy having a drink every now and then, does this mean you need to stop that, too?

It all depends. How severe is your acid reflux, and which foods or drinks tend to cause problems for you personally, in what amounts, and during what time of day are you most susceptible?

The National Heartburn Alliance (NHBA) Weighs In!

The National Heartburn Alliance developed a guide that names the specific foods in each food group/category that are the most likely to cause you trouble. Here are the highlights:

- **Meats and beans:** ground beef, marbled sirloin, chicken nuggets, and chicken/buffalo wings.
- **Fats, oils, and sweets:** chocolate, regular corn chips and potato chips, high-fat butter cookies, brownies, donuts, creamy and oily salad dressings, and liquor, wine, coffee, and tea.
- **Fruits and vegetables:** orange juice, lemon, lemonade, grapefruit juice, cranberry juice, tomato, mashed potatoes, French fries, raw onion, and potato salad.

- **Grains:** macaroni and cheese, spaghetti with marinara sauce.
- **Dairy:** sour cream, milk shakes, ice cream, regular cottage cheese.

For more information from the NHBA, visit their Website at *www.heartburnalliance.org*

Q: Why do I have heartburn every time I eat spicy foods?

I don't know if you noticed, but spicy foods (other than chili peppers and pepper) aren't anywhere to be found in the lists above. That's because they don't actually cause heartburn. They just make you more aware of it, which definitely counts in my book. In other words, eating spicy food isn't going to increase the acid in your stomach or suddenly weaken your esophageal sphincter muscle, but when this happens and the stomach contents come in contact with the esophagus, the presence of the spices will help irritate the esophagus.

Q: What do I do if I love spicy foods?

- Eat spicy foods in small portions.
- Avoid eating a large meal at the same time you have your small amount of spicy food (overeating in general can exaggerate heartburn).
- Try not to wash your little spicy meal down with alcohol or coffee (even decaf).
- Try not to take a nap or lie down for several hours after your little spicy meal.
- Chew some gum after the meal to help increase the flow of saliva.

Q: What are some alternatives to spicy condiments?

Some people tolerate small amounts of cider and rice vinegar, but here are some other condiments with which some people have no trouble: soy sauce, mustard, honey mustard, light mayonnaise, and fruit spreads. And in general, dried spices and herbs are less likely to promote heartburn, including dried onion and garlic, ground cinnamon, mace, ground ginger, coriander, dill, basil, thyme, cumin, and tarragon. Two of my favorite fresh herbs, basil and cilantro, are thought to be well tolerated. So find the dried spices and herbs that you can tolerate, and keep them handy when cooking!

Q: Alcohol—too much of a good thing?

Some studies have actually shown that small amounts of alcohol may actually protect the mucosal layer. It is also known that a low dose of alcohol accelerates gastric emptying; this can be a good thing when you have acid reflux. The sooner your stomach empties its meal into the small intestine, the sooner your esophagus isn't being tormented by the stomach contents.

But that is where alcohol helping acid reflux ends. Alcohol relaxes the sphincter muscle (potentially encouraging acid reflux) and it can also irritate the mucous membrane of the esophagus as it is going down. In terms of digestion, you can get too much of a good thing, too. Whereas a low dose of alcohol can speed stomach emptying in the small intestine, high doses of alcohol slow stomach emptying (almost as if the stomach is confused and drunk), and slows the movement of the bowel (*Am. J. Gastroenterology,* 95 (2000): 3374-82).

How much is a little? It really depends on the person. Some of the people to whom I spoke were able to manage their symptoms with no more than one drink a day.

Which types of alcohol are we talking about? All types of alcohol are suspect, although some people mentioned a particular problem with red wine.

Q: If I switch to decaf coffee can I still have it?

The roasted coffee beans that make coffee contain proteins that actually promote stomach acid secretion. Decaf coffee has these proteins just as much as regular coffee beans do. So, although switching to decaf may help with other health problems, it probably won't cure your acid reflux ills. But look for "easy on the stomach" coffees, which may or may not help you personally. Most of these are low-acid coffees being sold under the brands: Simply Smooth (Folgers), Gentle Java (Coffee Legends), and Puroast Low Acid Coffee.

Sometimes it isn't the quality of food—it's the quantity

Even if you follow the rules and stay away from foods that tend to aggravate your acid reflux, you could very well find your symptoms are still fast and furious. This could be because you aren't looking at the quantity of food you are eating. The more you eat, the more of a load it will be for your stomach, and the longer those contents will be churning away in your stomach. Eating small, frequent meals through the day and eating light at night is a great way to eat for many health reasons (better for diabetes, obesity, etc.), so now you can add acid reflux to the list. There's a food step to freedom devoted just to this novel and healthful way of eating. You can read more about it, starting on page 59.

If your bedtime is 10 p.m., the last call for dinner should be 6 p.m.

Late night meals are a problem. Lying down shortly after you eat or drink is asking for trouble. The reason is purely physical; when you are standing or sitting up, your stomach is upright and the stomach contents have to work against gravity to splash up into your esophagus. But when you lie down or recline, the stomach contents automatically churn against the valve separating the upper stomach from the lower esophagus, because gravity is no longer holding it back.

To make sure your last meal has mostly left the stomach by the time you are ready to go to sleep, avoid eating or drinking for at least three or four hours before lying down. This means if bedtime is 10 p.m., the last call for dinner should be around 6 p.m. While we are at it, it is also a good idea not to exercise vigorously soon after eating, particularly activities involving bending or running, which also encourages refluxing.

Q: Are there any foods or habits that are heartburn "helpers"?

Saliva to the rescue!

When it comes to acid reflux, saliva is a "good thing." Saliva, which is alkaline, helps bathe the lower esophagus, providing a little protection from the refluxing stomach acid. What can you do after a meal to increase your saliva and reduce the severity of heartburn?

- Chew gum (bubble gum or non-citrus fruit flavors).
- Suck on antacids or lozenges.
- Eat sweet pickles.

Got Gum?

The saliva stimulated by chewing seems to help neutralize acid and force stomach fluids back where it belongs—the stomach!

In one study, when 31 people were given heartburn-inducing meals and then some of the participants were told to chew sugar-free gum for 30 minutes, they found the acid levels in the esophagus to be significantly lower in gum chewers.

Another study noticed heartburn suppression benefits of post-meal gum chewing could last up to three hours!

Eating slowly

Relax. Take your time eating your meals and snacks. You are less likely to eat a large amount of food at one sitting when you take your time and enjoy every bite. Eating meals that are smaller in size and calories help you avoid heartburn.

Eating small and frequently

Eating smaller, more frequent meals throughout the day and eating light at night is a great eating style for many health reasons, including acid reflux. For more on this, along with holiday tips and recipes to help you avoid heartburn, see Chapter 3.

Q: Can you walk and chew at the same time?

Chewing gum for one hour after a meal can reduce the time that stomach acid is in contact with the esophagus, according to a new study by the department of Veterans Affairs Medical Center in New Mexico (*Aliment. Pharmacol. Ther.,* 15 (2001):151-5).

Chapter 3

The 10 Food Steps to Freedom

Q: Does the title "The 10 Food Steps to Freedom" mean that if I do these 10 things I will be totally free of acid reflux?

I wish the answer was yes, but unfortunately it's no. The 10 Food Steps to Freedom means, if you put together the most important food-and lifestyle-related tips you have read so far in this book, you arrive at 10 food/lifestyle steps to bring you closer to freedom from acid reflux symptoms.

This reminds me of that joke that always begins, "Doctor, every time I do _____, I'm in pain and agony," to which the doctor replies, "then don't do _____." Just fill in the blank with your own food—the one diet habit that sends you into heartburn hell. Something like, "Doctor, every time I eat greasy, deep fried food, I get heartburn something awful!" To which the doctor replies, "Then don't eat greasy, deep fried food!"

Everybody's acid reflux is different. Some people have milder symptoms and less esophageal damage, while others could have more severe symptoms or more advanced damage to their esophagus. Some people find that certain foods and drinks give them problems, while others say it's the amount of food and time of day that matters most. Some people battle heartburn during the day hours, while others suffer mainly at night.

The bottom line is that diet does not directly cause acid reflux. But acid reflux can be encouraged and aggravated by food and drink.

Step 1: Eat frequent, small meals instead of less-frequent big meals

Food Step

There's two ways to look at this food step. You can either look at it as eating smaller, more frequent meals, or you can look at it as avoiding eating *big* meals. Americans tend to do the opposite of this food step—we may skip a meal or two, but when we eat, we tend to eat *big*. This is a tough habit to break. The key to eating small, frequent meals for me is keeping this basic belief in check: Eat when you are hungry and stop when you are comfortable.

In my experience, when we do this, we automatically end up eating smaller-sized meals, which means we get hungry sooner, so we end up eating more often.

Eating more often, but smaller amounts at a time, is a good idea for every American, for a variety of sound health reasons, but it can be particularly helpful for people with acid reflux. Here's why:

- Smaller, lower fat meals don't stay in the stomach as long as larger, higher fat meals; they move more quickly to the intestines. And the shorter the time food is waiting around in the stomach, the shorter the time the stomach contents (including the stomach acid) are potentially splashing around, irritating the upper GI.

- Large meals fill up the stomach and are more likely to put pressure on the lower esophageal sphincter to open, allowing the contents of the full stomach to splash up into the esophagus. Picture an empty 2-liter soda bottle with 2 cups of liquid in it, screw on the top, and agitate the liquid. It is fairly difficult to get the liquid to splash around and hit the bottle cap isn't it? Now, fill that same 2-liter soda bottle with 6 cups of liquid. Suddenly hitting that bottle cap with some of the liquid is a lot easier now that the bottle is almost full. Your stomach acts much the same way.

Q: What is it about large meals that encourages heartburn?

Is it the volume of food in the stomach? Is it the amount of calories? A recent study from Germany (*Aliment Pharmacol. Ther.,* Feb. 2001; 15[2]: 233-9) tried to answer those questions. They concluded that the amount of acid reflux induced by eating a meal seemed to depend more on the volume of food rather than the density of calories in the meal. In other words, these researchers are suggesting that if you ate enough of almost anything, even if it was low in calories, it could quite possibly encourage heartburn because of the amount you ate.

Other amazing benefits of "eating small"

If you don't want to eat small, frequent meals through the day to help your acid reflux, then do it for these other great reasons:

- Your brain and body require a constant supply of energy in the blood. Eating smaller, more frequent meals is more likely to keep your blood sugar and energy level stable, which can prevent headaches, ir-ritability, food cravings, or overeating in susceptible people.

- The bigger the meal, the larger the number of calories eaten from carbohydrates, fat, and protein, and the higher the blood levels of those nutrients will be after the "large" meal. Large meals also zap you of your after-meal energy. If you've had a large meal, a nap is usually not far behind. But if you eat smaller meals you will feel more energetic throughout your day.

- It's physically more comfortable to eat smaller meals. You aren't weighed down by a large meal in your stomach. If you feel "light" on your feet, you will also be more likely to be physically active, too. And the more physically active you are, the more calories you will burn during the day, which helps you stay trim and shed those extra pounds around the middle...which reduces your acid reflux symptoms!

- Eating smaller, more frequent meals is great for appetite control. The more stable blood sugars keep you from getting overly hungry, which can lead to overeating or making high-sugar or high-fat food choices.

- One study observed that obesity was less common in people who ate more frequent meals. People who eat smaller, more frequent meals are less likely to overeat at any meal. Larger meals flood your bloodstream with fat, protein, and carbohydrate calories. Your body has to get rid of any extra calories. What does this have to do with being overweight? All extra calories can be converted to body fat for energy storage.

- This is still being investigated, but it is possible that this eating style may help lower serum cholesterol. It stands to reason that, by avoiding large meals, you also prevent quick rises of serum triglycerides that typically follow large, fatty meals.

- We burn more calories digesting, absorbing, and metabolizing food just by eating more often. The body burns calories when it digests and absorbs food. Every time we eat, the digestion process kicks in. If we eat six small meals instead of two large ones, we start the digestive process three times more often every single day—burning more calories. Calories burned by activating the metabolism can amount to about five to 10 percent of the total calories we eat in a day.

Q: How frequent should the "smaller" meals be?

Experts have not yet determined the ideal eating pattern for people with acid reflux, but so far it seems that the closer together the meals are, the better the results. The longer the gap between a previous meal or snack and dinner, for example, the larger the dinner typically ends up being.

If you eat a small breakfast, a midmorning snack, a light lunch, then an afternoon snack, and a light dinner and maybe a nighttime snack, it adds up to six small meals for the day. Until researchers know more, the best advice I can give you is to space your meals according to your individual schedule, when you tend to get hungry.

Fight the urge to splurge at night

We burn 70 percent of our calories as fuel during the day, but when do many Americans eat the majority of their calories? During the evening hours. Eating small meals can break this habit. If you eat small meals throughout the day, eat when you're hungry and stop when you're comfortable, it should be easier to avoid eating large dinners and evening desserts and snacks. Keep in mind that what you eat in the evening will be hitting your blood stream pretty much around the time you are getting into your jammies. It isn't as though you are eating to fuel a marathon or anything.

Easier said than done

Our whole society is based on three meals a day—with dinner typically being the largest meal of the day. This is a hard habit to break. If you eat out often, it becomes particularly difficult not to eat a large meal. It requires extra diligence at restaurants to eat only half your meal and save the rest for later. If you are having spaghetti, you could eat the salad and half your entrée, then have the garlic bread and the rest of your spaghetti later or the next day. I'm not saying it isn't going to be difficult, but it can be done.

> **Keep your stomach comfortable, not full**
> *A stomach full of food is more likely to splash up into the esophagus, so filling up your stomach is simply more likely to give you heartburn.*

Food Step

Step 2: Lose some extra weight (if you are overweight), but not by fad dieting

There are those dreaded words again—"lose some extra weight." Don't you just hate it? Everyone always says it like it is so easy. Believe me, I know it's not.

Here's the thing though: Being overweight often worsens acid reflux symptoms, and many overweight people find relief from their acid reflux symptoms when they lose some weight.

The heartburn payoff may come sooner than you think, too. A recent study found that when overweight people with acid reflux participated in a healthy weight loss program, their reflux improved three weeks *before* their weight started to change. Instant gratification can be a very good thing!

If you are a woman with a Body Mass Index (BMI) above 30 (classified as obese), you have three times the risk of suffering from acid reflux, according to the Nurses' Health Study. But losing weight without falling for fad diets is such a complicated subject that I devoted Chapter 4 to it. (Keep in mind that anyone considering a weight loss and exercise program should have a thorough medical examination before they begin.)

> **Food Step**
>
> *Step 3: Avoid eating high-fat meals when possible to encourage weight loss (if appropriate) and to reduce acid reflux symptoms*

Fried or fatty foods are thought to weaken the lower esophageal sphincter muscle, which encourages acid reflux, and that's why the recommendation to avoid fried or fatty foods appears in many food guidelines given to people with acid reflux. It has also been reported that relaxation of the esophageal muscle tends to occur after meals, and that a fair amount of food fat in the small intestines appears to stimulate this reaction (*New England Journal of Medicine*, 331 (1994): 656).

But this food recommendation is under fire lately by some researchers who are questioning whether it is the volume of food or caloric density that is really causing problems.

Q: Do high-fat foods really wreak havoc?

Whether people with acid reflux should continue to avoid those greasy, creamy, high-fat foods is being hotly debated around the globe. Some researchers say experience shows that many high-fat foods cause big problems for some people. Some researchers say it's the volume of the meal, not the fat. Others still say it's the density of calories that really does the harm.

Could it possibly be all of the above? Or are there other, more subtle ways that fatty foods encourage heartburn in some people?

These ways could include the fact that the higher the fat content of the meal, the longer it tends to stay in the stomach before moving on to the small intestine. Or is it that we tend to overdo our favorite greasy, high-fat foods, leading the meal toward a high volume of food or a high caloric density?

In a recent article (*Eur. J. Gastroenterol. Hepatol.* 12 (2000): 1343-5), an Italian researcher stated that suggest that fatty meals, compared to balanced meals, do not promote acid reflux as long as the calorie load is the same. But a high-fat meal is more likely to contain the mother load of calories simply because every gram of fat is worth nine calories compared to a gram of carbohydrate and a gram of protein, which are each worth four calories.

I've literally lightened hundreds of recipes throughout the past 15 years. I have modified the fat by using reduced-fat ingredients, cutting out some of the fat that isn't absolutely needed, or replacing a fatty ingredient with something much lower in fat and calories. In every single case, there are always fewer calories after I cut the fat in half. Same dish, same amount of food in the serving, just half the fat and fewer calories.

If you want to go by the results of the recent study mentioned earlier, which concluded that it was the volume of the meal rather than the caloric density that influenced acid reflux, then what does that mean for fatty foods? I think of it this way: What types of foods do we tend to overeat? Do we overeat yogurt? Or steamed broccoli? Or grilled salmon? Last I checked, we tend to overeat foods such as French fries, pizza, ribs, steak, chocolate chip cookies, or chocolate cake—all notorious high-fat foods.

One of the other big reasons I suggest limiting portions of high-fat foods is because people tend to lose weight and keep it off if they aren't eating a high-fat diet. This is an important point, because one of the food steps to freedom is to lose excess weight (if overweight). So either way, it's probably a good idea to try choosing reduced-fat options when possible. For tips on eating less fat when eating out or eating in check out Chapters 6 and 7 and my latest books, *Food Synergy; Fry Light, Fry Right;* and *Comfort Food Makeovers.*

Food Step

Step 4: Foods and beverages that weaken the lower esophageal sphincter muscle should be eaten in very small portions or limited:

- Fried or fatty foods
- Chocolate
- Peppermint and spearmint
- Garlic
- Onions

The following drinks are considered to be inciting agents (they encourage acid reflux) and they should be limited, particularly before bed.

- Coffee (including decaffeinated coffee, which increases the acid content in the stomach)
- Caffeinated tea and cola drinks (increase acid content in the stomach)
- Alcoholic beverages

It's hard to believe something as refreshing as peppermint can cause trouble, but a known side effect to peppermint oil is heartburn, according to the National Center for Complementary and Alternative Medicine.

There is going to be a huge range of experiences with the previously mentioned foods. I spoke with many acid reflux sufferers and they all had different stories to tell. Some had no reaction or problem with garlic and onions, and others said they literally can't touch them from dinner on, or they suffer by nightfall. One man could have one cup of coffee first thing in the morning, but that was it. One women swore that drinking decaf herbal tea in the morning seemed to help her acid reflux.

What about alcohol? Does it matter what type of alcohol? Does it matter how much? Again, it depends. Some say red wine gives them the most grief. One man said one beer was his limit. My guess is anything with alcohol in it can weaken the sphincter muscle and encourage reflux if you have enough. Your job, should you choose to accept it, is to find out how much is too much for you. Some people find it easier not to have any alcohol at all.

Q: What's left to drink?

Sodas can bloat the abdomen, which increases the pressure in the stomach, encouraging the stomach acid to splash up into the esophagus. Tomato and citrus juices can irritate a damaged esophagus. Alcoholic beverages, coffee (even decaf) and caffeinated tea and cola can increase the acid content in the stomach, as well as relax the LES (lower esophageal sphincter muscle). So what's left? You could try water, mineral water without flavor essence or carbonation, decaffeinated green or black tea, non-citrus fruit juices, non-tomato vegetable juices, or skim and low-fat milk.

The chocolate clause

I can't imagine a day going by without a little bite of chocolate. I usually have my daily "bite" right after lunch. Don't ask me why, that's just when my body tells me its time. A bite could be a "fun size" Snickers bar or a small handful of chocolate chips. It's not a lot—just enough. So I would have a big problem with the previous list of foods to limit including my one favorite treat. One friend with acid reflux did okay with a small handful of M&Ms

but noticed discomfort anytime she had brownies. I asked the medical experts. Does it matter what type of chocolate? Does it matter how much chocolate? No one seemed to know—cocoa versus baker's chocolate, milk versus semi-sweet. How could they not know the answer to this very important question?

You will have to figure out for yourself what your chocolate clause is. Is a small handful fine, but more than that is off limits? Or is it that certain rich chocolate desserts (such as brownies) mean trouble. And does it help if the chocolate dessert is lower in fat?

Food Step

Step 5: Foods that increase the acid content of the stomach should be consumed in small portions

- Coffee (including decaffeinated coffee, which increases the acid content in the stomach).
- Caffeinated tea and cola drinks (increase acid content in the stomach).
- Calcium in milk. (It has been suggested that the calcium in milk increases stomach acid secretion.)

Reading this list is a little like déjà vu, because the same beverages were just listed in Step 4 as items that weaken the lower esophageal sphincter. Well, they also increase the acid content of the stomach. They are a double whammy when it comes to acid reflux. Some of you might find you can tolerate certain amounts of them at certain times of the day. Some people are going to be more sensitive during the day hours, while others can tolerate a cup of coffee first thing in the morning, but not late at night. You probably already know from experience when you are most likely to tolerate one little cup of coffee.

Food Step

Step 6: Foods that irritate a damaged esophageal lining should be limited (if your lining is damaged)

- Citrus fruits and citrus juices
- Tomatoes and tomato products
- Pepper
- Chili pepper (There is some research data that a phytochemical in chili pepper, capsaicin, may increase the sensitivity of the esophageal lining.)

Depending on the type of cuisine you favor, one or all of the previous foods is going to be rather tough to temper. If you find you have discomfort with tomatoes and tomato products, and you love Mexican and Italian foods, it's not going to be easy. If you find that chili pepper seems to bring on the heartburn and you enjoy eating Mexican and spicy Asian dishes, you aren't going to be happy either. You might be extremely sensitive and need to totally avoid the food, or you may find that a small amount, a virtual "taste" of it, is as far as you can go. You may even find you can have small amounts of these kinds of foods as long as they are earlier in the day (say, lunchtime) rather than later.

Q: Trouble spices?

The following spices may irritate the stomach lining:

- Black pepper
- Crushed red pepper
- Tabasco
- Chili powder
- Curry powder
- Mint
- Cloves
- Mustard seed

- Nutmeg
- Fresh garlic (raw or cooked)

Food Step	## Step 7: Foods that can bloat up the abdomen causing pressure that forces acid to back up into the esophagus should be limited

All carbonated beverages are to blame. I would personally have a hard time never drinking a carbonated beverage again. I'm one of those Diet-Pepsi-a-day drinkers. And man, am I ready for my Diet Pepsi by mid-afternoon! For many people, this food step is going to translate into limiting soda and carbonated beverages—not cutting them out completely. You may find that one soda in the afternoon goes down just fine. But a soda, after a fairly full meal late into the evening, may not.

Crazy over capsaicin? The pleasure and pain principle

There's a fine line between pleasure and pain. And depending on your taste buds and preferences, you may actually crave irritating ingredients such as chili peppers. Capsaicin is the primary pungent and irritating ingredient in chili peppers and red peppers, which are widely used as spices around the globe. Capsaicin elicits burning pain by activating specific receptors on sensory nerve endings. Either you think it hurts so good or you think it's all bad; that's if you don't have acid reflux.

If you do suffer from heartburn, capsaicin can actually do a number on you, above and beyond its usual irritating or pleasurable "hot" effect in your mouth. It's possible that capsaicin increases the sensitivity of the esophagus lining, making it particularly painful when stomach acid refluxes up beyond the esophageal muscle sphincter. We'll know more in years to come, but in the meantime when it comes to chili peppers, eat them at your own risk!

Step 8: Include high-fiber foods in every meal and snack

Food Step

Eat a high-fiber diet and help your heartburn? That's right—a recent study found that people who followed a high-fiber meal plan were 20 percent less likely to have acid reflux symptoms, regardless of their body weight. You'll find fiber in whole grains, fruits, vegetables, beans, nuts, and seeds (basically plant foods that we haven't done anything to). (*Gut*, January 2005, News Release, Dept. of Veterans Affairs "Dietary Intake and the risk of Gastroesophageal Reflux Disease" El-Serag, H.B.)

One of the most important steps to "including high fiber foods in every meal" is definitely switching to whole grains whenever possible. Here's why: a Dutch study looked at men and women between the ages of 55 and 69 and found as whole grain consumption went up, the body mass index (BMI) and the risk of overweight and obesity, went down (European Journal of Clinical Nutrition Sept. 26, 2007 Van de Vijver et al., "Whole-grain consumption, dietary fiber intake and body mass index in the Netherlands cohort study").

Count on fiber!

Getting enough fiber is something people don't usually think about all that often. Most of us haven't a clue about how many grams of fiber we are taking in on a typical day. The truth is, for many Americans, this number should be doubled!

According to a recent position paper by the American Dietetic Association on the Health Implications of Dietary Fiber, most of us aren't even coming close to the recommended intakes of 20–35 grams of fiber a day. The mean fiber intake in the United States is only half this amount—14 to 15 grams a day. It's not so surprising that these recommended fiber amounts are generally not being met when you think about which foods contribute fiber. We get fiber when we eat unprocessed plant foods such as fruits, vegetables, whole grains, nuts, seeds, beans, and the typical American isn't exactly loading their plates with these particular foods. You would be hard-pressed, for example, to find a fruit, vegetable, whole grain, or a bean in your average fast food value meal.

How Much Fiber Do We Need?

Recommended Fiber Intake: 25 g per day for a 2,000 calories a day diet.

Nutrition Facts labels: 30 g per day for a 2,500 calories a day diet.

All types of fiber are important

There's a difference between the type of fiber in wheat bran and lettuce and the type of fiber in oats and apples. One is generally a scrubbing type of fiber (not soluble in water) and one is a softer, thickening (viscous) type of fiber that binds with water. Both boast health benefits in the body.

Type of fiber: The softer fiber that binds with water (soluble or viscous).

How it benefits the body: It forms a gel-like material when it is digested that:

- Helps prevents cholesterol and saturated fats from entering the bloodstream, where they can collect and form plaques on artery walls. "The value of oat bran and its beta-glucan (soluble fiber) content in reducing several risk factors for cardiovascular disease is already well established," notes Dr. Jeffrey Blumberg, PhD, director of the Antioxidants Research Laboratory at Tufts University.

- This type of fiber is also thought to help minimize the rise in blood sugar levels after a meal, which can be particularly helpful for people with diabetes.

Food Sources: beans (have both types), oats and oat bran, barley, psyllium, some fruits (apples, mango, plums, kiwi, pears, blackberries, strawberries, raspberries, peaches, citrus fruits, dried apricots, prunes, and figs), and some vegetables (artichokes, celery root, sweet potato, parsnip, turnip, acorn squash, potato with skin, Brussels sprouts, cabbage, green peas, broccoli, carrots, French-style green beans, cauliflower, asparagus, and beets).

Type of fiber: Scrubbing fiber (that doesn't bind with water).

How it benefits the body: It helps keep bowel movements regular and may help reduce risk of colon problems. It may also reduce the risk of hemorrhoids, varicose veins, and obesity (by making us feel full).

Food Sources: Whole wheat and wheat bran, brown rice, bulgur, beans (have both types), the fruits and vegetables (in general) not listed previously for soluble fiber.

Q: Why is fiber so good for us?

It's hard to believe that something we can't even digest and absorb can be so good for us! Double your daily fiber totals and this is what you have to look forward to:

- Less heartburn.
- It helps slow digestion, which can help you eat less and lose weight (both of which can also help make heartburn less likely).
- Lower blood cholesterol levels.
- Improve and prevent constipation.

Fiber has been shown to increase satiety not only by lowering the energy density of foods, but also by slowing the rate that foods pass through the digestive tract. Simply doubling the amount of fiber you eat from the average of 15 grams per day to around 30 grams can help reduce calorie intake.

Dr. Joanne Slavin, PhD, an obesity researcher with the University of Minnesota, agrees that epidemiological studies continue to show the importance of high-fiber intakes and lower body weight. "The best protection is at the highest fiber intakes—at least 25 grams/day recommended for women," says Dr. Slavin. According to Dr. Slavin, dietary fiber makes us feel fuller, reduces digestibility, and helps regulate blood glucose and insulin, all reasons that people on higher fiber diets weigh less and are less prone to gain weight with age.

The 6 quickest ways to 25 grams of fiber

So how do we get more fiber into our daily diet quickly and painlessly? Here are six ways to work that fiber into your daily diet.

Get Those Whole Grains:
- 2 slices of whole wheat bread = 4 grams of fiber
- 1 cup of cooked brown rice = 4 grams of fiber
- 7 Reduced Fat Triscuit crackers = 3 grams

Breakfast Cereals:
- 1 cup of Raisin Bran = 7.5 grams of fiber
- 1 cup of Quaker Squares Baked in Cinnamon = 5 grams
- 1 cup of Frosted Shredded Wheat Spoonsize = 5 grams
- 3/4 cup of cooked oatmeal = 3 grams of fiber

Beans:

- 1 cup of canned minestrone soup = about 5 grams
- 1/2 cup of vegetarian or fat free refried beans = about 6 grams of fiber
- 1/4 cup of kidney beans added to green salads = 3 grams of fiber
- A bean burrito = 8 grams

Fruits:

You can add fruit to your morning meal, enjoy fruit as a snack, and garnish your dinner plate with some fun fruit. You can even have fruit with or instead of dessert.

- 1 large apple = 4 grams of fiber
- 1 banana = 3 grams of fiber
- 1 pear = 4 grams of fiber
- 1 cup of strawberries = 4 grams of fiber

Flaxseed: A tablespoon a day into your smoothie, cup of soup, casserole serving, and so on. Just those two tablespoons will boost your daily fiber total by 6 grams! Flaxseed contains a balance of soluble and insoluble fiber too.

Veggies: Work them in any way you can, and try to get several servings every single day. Include a vegetable with lunch, have raw vegetables as an afternoon snack or pre-dinner appetizer, and enjoy a big helping of vegetables with dinner. You can even make a point of enjoying vegetarian entrees several times a week or more.

- 1 cup carrot slices, cooked = 5 grams of fiber
- 1 cup cooked broccoli = 4.5 grams of fiber
- 1 cup raw carrots = 4 grams of fiber
- 1 sweet potato = 4 grams of fiber
- 1 cup cauliflower, cooked = 3 grams of fiber
- 2 cups raw spinach leaves = 3 grams of fiber

Fiber All-Stars

Food	Fiber (in grams)
Bran cereal, 1/2 cup	10
Beans, lentils, 1/2 cup	6–9
Artichoke, 1 medium	6.5
Spaghetti, whole-wheat, 1 cup	6
Pear, 1 medium	5
Rye (whole rye) crackers, 2	5
Sweet potato, 1 medium	5
Peas, green, frozen, 1/2 cup	5
Whole wheat bread, 2 slices	4–8
Blackberries/raspberries, 1/2 cup	4
Oat bran, 1/4 cup	4
Popcorn, 6 cups	4
Potato, baked, 1 medium	4
Prunes, stewed, 1/2 cup	4
Vegetables, mixed, cooked, 1/2 cup	4
Apple, large	1
Broccoli, 1 cup cooked	6
Almonds, 1 ounce	3.5
Spinach, 1/2 cup cooked or 2 cups raw	3.5
Banana, 1 medium	3
Orange, 1 medium	3
Strawberries, whole, 1 cup	3

Words to the wise

- When fiber is increased, water intake should increase along with it!

- When increasing fiber, do it gradually to give your gastro-intestinal tract time to adapt.

- Caution should be used when recommending fiber to those with gastrointestinal diseases, including constipation. Just check with your doctor first before going out of your way to boost your fiber.

Food Step

Step 9: Don't eat three to four hours before going to bed

Put another way, don't lie down up to four hours after eating. Back in Chapter 1, we talked about how when you lie down your body becomes horizontal instead of vertical, which means your stomach suddenly becomes horizontal too. And if there is anything substantial in your stomach when you do lie down, it has a better chance of splashing up (refluxing) than if the stomach was right side up. When you are sitting upright, the stomach content has to work against gravity to splash up into the lower esophagus.

For more advice on how to sleep with acid reflux, check out the tips toward the end of Chapter 1.

The bewitching hour

The interesting thing is there is a significant number of acid reflux sufferers who actually have less of a problem at night, and actually have more trouble during the day hours. Most people, however, find that the bewitching hours are the ones that usually follow dinner.

| Food Step | ***Step 10: Have your heartburn helpers handy and make other lifestyle changes that can help your heartburn*** |

Here are four helpful lifestyle changes you can make today:

1. Have your hearburn helpers handy. The following foods and activities help by increasing saliva. The bicarbonate in saliva helps neutralize the acid and the thickness of saliva helps bathe your esophagus lining, providing a slight buffer to incoming stomach acid.

   - Chewing gum (fruit-flavored or bubble gum instead of mint—if mint seems to be a trigger for you) after meals stimulates saliva production. Chew gum after meals also increases peristalsis (the waves of involuntary muscle contractions that transport food through the GI tract), which helps move the stomach contents into the small intestine more quickly.

   - Sucking on antacids or lozenges after meals stimulates saliva production.

   - Drinking plain old tap water may help dilute the acid in your stomach and help remove acid that is coating the esophagus. When you drink a small glass of water at the end of your meals, it helps dilute and wash down any stomach acid that might be splashing up into the esophagus.

   - Eating sweet pickles (has been suggested by some to help).

2. Keep a heartburn journal to get a better idea of what is encouraging heartburn. Write down what you are eating, when you are eating, and how much you are eating, and keep track of when heartburn is striking. See if you can find any clues or patterns.

Keeping a heartburn and food journal

The truth is that each person has his or her own heartburn triggers. There are certainly some common denominators—and we talk about them all through this book—but it really helps to know what is triggering your heartburn, be it specific foods or beverages you eat or drink in certain amounts at certain times of day. You can usually identify your food and beverage triggers a lot better if you make an effort to jot it down in a heartburn/food log.

Here's a sample page to get an idea of what you could write down each day. If you have heartburn, write down in the "Heartburn" column when the heartburn started, and how severe the pain was. If you take medication, write down what you took and at what time.

Day 1	Date:		
Time Food/Drink	Heartburn (how bad)?	Medication
6 a.m.			
8 a.m.			
10 a.m.			
12 p.m.			
2 p.m.			
4 p.m.			
6 p.m.			
8 p.m.			
10 p.m.			

3. Stop smoking! Smoking weakens the lower espophageal sphincter (LES) muscle between the upper stomach and lower esophagus.
4. Elevate the head of the bed 6 inches.

A sample heartburn-free day

Reading the diet suggestions in the food steps to freedom can be daunting and hard to visualize. Here is a sample day that ties together most of the suggestions, so you can see how it all might fit together for you.

6:30 a.m. breakfast

- High-fiber hot or cold cereal with nonfat or 1-percent low-fat milk.
- Low fat turkey bacon.
- Apple or grape juice.

10 a.m. morning snack

- Container low-fat yogurt.
- 1/2 cup fresh fruit.
- Decaf green tea.

12:30 p.m. lunch

- Roasted turkey and avocado sandwich on whole wheat bread.
- Baby carrots or other raw veggies.
- End the meal with a glass of water.
- Chew some fruit-flavored or bubble gum after the meal instead of mint-flavored gum.

3:30 p.m. afternoon snack

- Whole grain crackers.
- Reduced fat cheese.
- Apple slices.
- Decaf green tea.

5:30–6:30 p.m. exercise/workout

7 p.m. dinner

- Higher fiber pasta (such as Barilla Plus).
- With pesto sauce or some lean meat or fish if desired (such as cooked shrimp or strips of lean beef).
- Steamed vegetables.
- A light dessert (such as frozen fruit bar).
- End the meal with a glass of water.
- Chew some non-peppermint gum after the meal.

10:30 p.m. bedtime

The bottom line

It isn't an exact science. It all basically comes down to what, when, and how much. *What* you eat, *how much* you eat, and *when* you eat can be helpful or hurtful for your particular acid reflux. The 10 Food Steps to Freedom show you what tends to bother most or some people, and helps explain how they encourage acid reflux. Beyond that, you have to write your own story about your own acid reflux.

Chapter 4

Waiting to Lose Weight

Why is there a whole chapter about losing weight in a book about acid reflux? Granted, you can have acid reflux and be as thin as a super model, but the truth is that the majority of people suffering from acid reflux are overweight. And the excess baggage (so to speak), especially when it's around the mid-portion, can exacerbate the acid reflux.

As little as a 10-percent drop in weight (if overweight or obese) can improve hearburn symptoms. Or, put another way, even moderate weight gain among normal-weight people may cause or exacerbate acid reflux symptoms.

Think about it: those 10 to 20 extra pounds around your belly are physically adding pressure to the stomach, which tends to push the stomach contents up toward the top of the stomach. This is generally not a good thing when you have acid reflux.

I'll tell you right now, I don't believe in fad dieting. It's simply one of the worst things you can do. First of all, the weight loss never lasts. Generally, there is only a 5-percent success rate when you look at maintained weight loss during a five-year period, and one-third gain it back by the one-year point. That means for every

100 people on these various diets, at best, only five people haven't gained the weight back five years down the line. Not only that, but any time you embark on a quick weight loss scheme, you are making it more difficult for your body to shed pounds in the future.

Each time you lose weight quickly, your body gets better and better at gaining and holding onto this extra weight the next time around. One of the reasons for this is because when you lose weight quickly, you tend to lose muscle/protein mass. But when the pounds come back on, they tend to come back as body fat. This loss in muscle decreases the amount of calories you burn maintaining your basic body functions. The less calories you burn just maintaining your body function, the more likely you will have extra calories and put on extra body weight.

Just say no to dieting and dieting products

I fully realize that staying away from dieting is an upward battle in this country. Every single day you are being overwhelmed by celebrities telling you how they stay thin, and articles in magazines telling you how to lose weight fast—each advising you that this is truly "the answer." Don't believe it. Resist the urge and just walk on by. In case you still have a few questions though, here are the questions people keep asking me about fad diets.

Do the high-protein, low-carbohydrate fad diets help you lose weight? Are there any risks?

Anytime a high-protein, low-carbohydrate eating plan is recommended it is not intended for long-term use. Carbohydrates, not protein, are the preferred fuel source for the body. When the body uses protein for energy, nitrogen must be removed first, and all the extra nitrogen must be removed from the body (via urine), because too much circulating in the blood is toxic. This can over-tax the kidneys. Anyone with impaired kidney function should not even attempt a high-protein diet.

Here's one weight loss fact you should always remember. Fat gets stored in the body when the calories we take in are higher than the calories we are burning—regardless of where those calories came from.

The long-term effects of high-protein fad diets have not been studied. It is true that many people will lose weight on these plans because they are mostly low calorie plans, and by limiting carbohydrate they are forcing the followers to limit portion size. The weight loss has more to do with the decrease in total calories and forced portion sizing, and less to do with the fact that it is high in protein. But how healthy and permanent the weight loss is on this plan remains to be proven. I have met several people who lost weight on one of these high-protein plans. None of them maintained the lost weight—each is back to where they started.

Q: Are high-protein diets more healthful than high-carbohydrate diets?

No! But the high-carbohydrate diet is hopefully nicely balanced with some protein and some fat, and features mostly complex carbohydrates (whole grains, vegetables, beans, and fruits) and not lots of sugar and refined grains. Don't forget there are many important nutrients in grains, fruits, vegetables, beans (carbohydrate-rich foods), such as fiber and phytochemicals, that are mostly absent in those high-protein plans. High-protein diets are often high in saturated fat, too. Most can't even follow them for more than a few months, because they are just too difficult to keep up. The bottom line is that there is no evidence that individuals who lose weight on such diets maintain their weight loss over people who lost it by eating a healthy, more balanced diet with lots of plant foods..

Q: Do high-protein diets help or hurt acid reflux?

My guess is they will hurt acid reflux, but the truth is we don't have the research to know that for sure. However, this is what we do know: When you eat a meal, the hormone gastrin, is released in the stomach, which stimulates the production of hydrochloric acid. Hydrochloric acid helps digest food as it enters the stomach, but the flip side to that is it is also the main acid involved in heartburn. There is something else in the food we eat that helps stimulate the release of gastrin (which stimulates hydrochloric acid), and that's protein. This is because one of the only major items being digested in the stomach is protein. This stomach acid uncoils the protein and begins to break down proteins into smaller units—amino acids.

So that's one big reason why a high-protein diet might not bode well for people with acid reflux. Here's another reason: many high-protein animal foods also contribute a big dose of fat and rich, high-fat meals are known to be a common heartburn trigger. But recently the National Heartburn Alliance did a small informal survey with people who responded that they had been on one of the low-carbohydrate diets. About half said their symptoms worsened or didn't change, while the other half said their symptoms greatly or slightly improved. The trouble with the survey is the low-carb diets followed ranged from the Atkins or South Beach diet to simply eating less bread and pasta.

Q: I keep hearing about carbohydrates, the addicts diet, refined, complex, simple—what do I need to know?

Don't be swayed by the carbohydrate-hating rhetoric out there. What is lost in the carbohydrate message is that there are different types of carbohydrates, and you just can't lump sugar in the same nutritional camp as broccoli or whole wheat bread—that's ridiculous. Certainly no one has evidence that we shouldn't be eating whole grains, beans, fruits, and vegetables. As for lots of soda, fat-free, high-sugar cookies, and processed grains, that's another story. Here are some definitions to help you sift through the information.

- **Simple carbohydrates:** Single sugar molecules or parts of sugar molecules bonded together. These single sugars are the building blocks for all carbohydrates. Naturally occurring sugars are glucose, fructose, or galactose. Table sugar is two sugars bonded together, sucrose and lactose, and the sugar found in milk, is also made of two sugars (glucose and galactose). Simple carbohydrates digest rapidly to form glucose molecules.

- **Complex carbohydrates:** Long strands of sugar molecules linked together. They take longer to break down to glucose. Breads, pastas, grain-based foods, and starchy vegetables such as potatoes and corn are excellent sources of complex carbohydrates.

- **Refined carbohydrates:** These have had certain components of the plant removed, usually the germ and bran. Both simple and complex carbohydrates can be "refined." Table sugar is refined from raw sugar. White flour is refined from whole-wheat grain. Even fruit juice is refined if some of the pulp and fiber has been removed.

It just makes sense to emphasize the complex, unrefined carbohydrates. They contain the germ of the grain, which contains essential vitamins and helpful oils, and the bran, which contributes fiber and phytochemicals. Generally, the higher the fiber in a carbohydrate, the more "complex" the carbohydrate, and the slower it converts from carbohydrate eaten to glucose in the blood, which helps most people maintain consistent blood sugar levels, at the very least.

Q: What about the advertisements I see for foods and products that help you burn fat while you sleep?

To burn body fat your body has to be in a deficit situation where it requires more calories than it is taking in with food. This means exercise, building muscle, and eating less than your body requires. You know what they say: if it sounds too good to be true, it usually is. Anybody can tell you anything to help sell a product. Most quick and fast claims have no real science backing them up.

You should also avoid buying weight-loss products using "speed" substances, such as ephedra, ma huang, guarana, or high doses of caffeine. These may artificially increase your metabolic rate, but can be absolutely dangerous. These substances don't offer any long-term weight-loss advantages, and that's what really matters. Try to avoid the temptation of a quick fix. Trimming off extra pounds takes time. Concentrate on eating healthy and exercising; this benefits your body in many different ways—trimming off extra weight is just one of them.

No one can go on these fad diets for very long, because you eventually get tired of it. And anytime you are "dieting" you are spending the bulk of your waking time and energy thinking about and following this new diet. Folks, that's not what life is supposed to be about, and eating should be about satisfying hunger, nourishing your body, and yes, even enjoying the meal.

Kill two heartburn birds with one stone (eat more fruits and vegetables!)

Eating more fruits and vegetables will help you with Food Step #2 (lose some extra weight if you are overweight, but not by fad dieting) and Food Step #8 (include high-fiber foods in every meal and snack).

If you are hoping for a secret weapon to jump-start your weight loss and help increase your fiber, you might want to point yourself in the direction of the nearest produce section. It's not quite as simple as just eating six or more servings of fruits and vegetables a day and watching the pounds melt away, but it's as good as it gets.

There are three reasons why fruits and vegetables should be considered secret weapons for weight loss:

- Most fruits and vegetables are high in water.
- Most fruits and vegetables are high in fiber.
- Most fruits and vegetables are low in calories.

For all three reasons, fruits and vegetables help give a feeling of fullness without the higher calories of foods that are higher in fat. And don't underestimate this potential power of produce! A recent study looked at what happens when you feed overweight people prepared meals that have more vegetables and fruits and are lower in fat than meals they normally eat. They had significant weight loss! In another study, when people ate more vegetables and fruits in meals, they reduced their total calorie consumption by more than 400 calories per day! That's pretty impressive for a couple of food groups that we should eat more of anyway to promote health and prevent disease.

You can sum up this power of produce in two words—energy density. Energy density is the relationship of calories to the volume of food (the three-dimensional space that a food takes up on your plate and in your stomach). For weight loss, foods that are low in energy density are good to include—these are foods that are low in calories for their volume or space. Makes sense, right?

Adding fruits and vegetables to your daily menu can theoretically reduce energy density, promote satiety, and decrease your food/calorie intake. There have been several studies looking specifically at the effect of increased weight loss by adding fruits and vegetables, and many have shown a definite benefit. In another study, the group that was told to increase fruits and vegetables lost more weight after one year than the group told to decrease fat and sugar. The trick seems to be substituting fruits and vegetables for high-energy, dense foods or adding in fruits and vegetables to meals so that the same volume is eaten as before, but the new produce-enriched meals are lower in calories.

Be careful about how you prepare and process fruits and vegetables

It's pretty obvious that fruits and vegetables are a great weight loss or weight maintenance tool. But does it matter how they are processed and prepared? You know the answer to this, don't you? A whole apple cut into wedges has more satiating power than pureed apples or fiber-free apple juice. The same can be said about oranges and orange juice or grapes and grape juice. So, remember to choose your fruits and vegetables with this in mind—the less processed the better.

We also have a habit of taking these naturally low-energy dense fruits and vegetables and adorning them with ingredients that can raise the energy density. I'm talking about dousing low-calorie green salads with high-fat and high-calorie salad dressings, cheese, and croutons, or smothering innocent sweet potatoes with butter and brown sugar.

Maintaining the joy of eating

Healthy food isn't going to do anyone any good if no one's eating it. Food should be enjoyed. With all this talk about what's good for our bodies, and what's not so good, that enjoyment part can sort of get lost in the nutritional shuffle. I don't want that to happen, because if it doesn't taste good, chances are, you won't be able to stick to your new healthy dietary habits for very long.

There is something less obvious that can zap the joy right out of eating: counting. Counting calories, fat grams, or tabulating food group servings—take your pick. If you have to count anything having to do with your food, it can take the joy not only out of eating, but also out of living. Anytime you put yourself in a "counting" mode, day in and day out, you automatically snap into the "dieting" mentality, which often leaves you feeling defeated, deprived, and depressed.

Don't get me wrong, I don't mind periodic counting. That's when, every now and then, you check in to see how your average daily food intake compares to certain standards or recommendations. It can be useful as long as it is a checkpoint and not a daily regimen. There are people who, for their continued health, have to count certain nutrients (people with diabetes or renal disease). Believe me, one of their greatest challenges is maintaining the joy of eating.

Beauty is in the eye of the beholder

In some parts of the world and in other points in history, my curvy and round size 14 figure would be considered very desirable. It was only until the early 1900s that the Rubenesque women painted by Rafael and Renoir (around the mid-to late-1800s) were no longer considered the female "ideal." In their time, extra weight on women was a sign of being rich and healthy.

It was in the early 1900s that corsets and the age of the thin flapper dancer became popular. Then in the mid-1900s curves seemed to be coming back in with Marilyn Monroe, a gorgeous and curvy size 14, leading the charge. Unfortunately today, many women are embarrassed to be a size 14.

Then the 1960s ushered in the age of miniskirts and bony women. I don't think we've shaken this yet, even after 30-plus years. Beauty contestants, models, and Hollywood actresses have never been thinner. To add confusion to the mix, obesity and eating disorders in this country have only been increasing. And yet, these past 20 years we have, as a nation, fed billions of dollars into the dieting business. For what? It hasn't worked. We've never been more unhappy and more obese. Why do we keep pumping more dollars into fad diets. Why aren't we pumping iron instead? Why do we hate our bodies? Why aren't we celebrating our curves and focusing on health and fitness instead?

Call me an optimist, but I think the pendulum is finally swinging back a smidgen. Finally there are more "normal"-sized women models, thanks to Emme and talk show hosts (such as some of the ladies on *The View*). And there are starting to be truly fashionable clothing stores and catalogues for women size 12 and up. It's like a breath of fresh air. I have recently noticed television specials on the new idea of "beauty" (which is probably really an "old" idea that's just coming back).

Just the other night I was watching a cable special on what men and women (past and present) are looking for in a mate. They interviewed men and women in parts of North Eastern Africa and the men in this particular village said they were looking for a wife who was strong, had wide hips, and could have many children. I remember thinking, hey, they're describing a curvaceous, and sturdy-framed person similar to myself.

You're not getting older, you're getting heavier

Marilyn Monroe aside, the sad truth is that as we age, body water, bone density, and muscle mass all tend to decrease while body fat increases. We can fight this by keeping our hydration and bone density as high as possible, and by maintaining and building our muscle mass as we age. Sounds simple, doesn't it? If it were *really* simple, more of us would be doing it, wouldn't we? Hopefully the following tips will make it as easy as possible.

Trade in those fad diets for fitness

Most experts and chronic dieters can agree on one thing—dieting doesn't work. When tempted by new diets out there, remember this—quick weight loss tends to break down lean body tissue (muscles and organ tissue). Weight regain tends to put on body fat—exactly the opposite of what we want to happen. And each time you lose weight and gain it back, the more difficult it's going to be to lose that weight again. If you've lost weight and gained it back several times, then you know exactly what I'm talking about.

If we could all change our goal from losing weight to gaining health, we would all be better off. To gain health, we simply focus on eating healthy and getting regular exercise. To help us do this, it is essential we remember two things:

1. You don't have to be thin to be fit and healthy.
2. A healthy weight is a fit weight (not considered in the "obese" range) that you maintain by eating healthy foods without overeating, fad dieting, or eating disorders.

Get in a "health" mindset

If you focus on losing pounds, you immediately put yourself in a dieting mindset where you are more likely to fall into the weighing-yourself-daily failure trap. Change your focus to being and feeling healthy. I believe in eating and exercising for the health of it, and let the pounds fall where they may.

> **Obesity isn't attributed to a lack of willpower anymore**
> *Obesity is now understood to result from a complex inter-action of genetic, metabolic, behavioral, and environmental factors.*

Don't give up just because you have the fat genes

We can't do anything about the genetic factors that influence obesity. On the other hand, we can't let our genes get in the way of our feeling good and being healthy. Your genes do enhance your susceptibility to gain weight in times of feast (versus famine), particularly when "feasting" with a high-fat diet. But if we eat a more healthful moderate fat diet, with lots of plant foods, and we get physically fit, we are going to temper our genetic pull toward overweight.

We can also work on some of the other factors that influence obesity—such as the behavioral and psychological factors that influence our particular lives. We can look at our eating habits and what might be triggering us to overeat at times. If it looks as if you have some issues with dieting, food, and body image, it might be a good idea to work with a psychologist or specially trained counselor to help you work through your particular past (so you can get on with your future). By the way, many people have long-standing issues with food, so please don't feel alone in this.

I know what it's like to have the fat gene on both sides of the family tree. My sisters and I have never been thin, but we were athletes through much of our youth, and that helped us concentrate on what really mattered—health.

Take inventory of your eating habits

The one area you might need to look at more closely is changing the habits that might be leading you to excess weight. Do you have any unhealthy habits? Take the quiz below and find out:

The "What's Your Habit?" Quiz

- Do you snack on sweets and chips more than fresh fruit and vegetables?

- Do you eat everything on your plate every time, thinking you would be wasting food if you didn't?

- Do you find yourself eating when you aren't really hungry because you are under stress, bored, angry, or upset? (Research indicates that using food to soothe feelings may be one big reason many people who lose weight gain it back.)

- Do you think you are being "bad" when you have your favorite foods? Do you think you must give them up in order to lose weight?

- Do you sometimes sit down for a small snack and end up eating a whole box of cookies, bag of chips, or small carton of ice cream?

- Do you sometimes let yourself get too hungry because you are trying to lose weight by not eating, even when you are hungry?

- Do you eat a lot of food late at night?

Now, trade in the destructive habits for the following healthful habits:

- Do you eat when you are hungry and stop when you are comfortable (not full)?

- Do you eat mostly plant foods, making sure you eat at least five servings of fruits and vegetables every day?

- Do you drink alcohol only on occasion (or not at all)? When you do drink, do you keep it at one drink a day?

- If there is a certain food you really want, and you are physically hungry, do you have it in a small but satisfying portion?

- Are you trying to eat more fiber-rich foods (fruits, vegetables, whole grains) and more balanced meals and snacks, including some protein and fat (mostly monounsaturated fat), because this generally makes meals more satisfying and staves off hunger longer?

- Do you eat light at night, knowing you will be more comfortable sleeping if you aren't full, waking up hungry, and ready to start your day?

- Do you exercise regularly because you know it is important for your overall health?

- Do you avoid distractions—such as reading or watching television—when you eat? Do you try to eat slowly and savor the taste of food?

- Do you find other ways to comfort yourself when you are bored, stressed, angry, or upset? (These activities could be things such as going for a walk, calling a friend, listening to some uplifting music, or taking a bubble bath.) Don't ignore your feelings—find healthier ways of dealing with them. It's easier said than done, but get professional counseling with this if you need it.

- Do you weigh yourself only when in doctor's offices because you know that the numbers on the scale really don't matter? What matters most is your overall health and how you feel.

Eat when you are hungry and stop when you are comfortable

This is a big key to nourishing yourself. Don't forget this. It's important. But think about it—everything about dieting goes against this. Dieting tells you not to listen to your hunger. When you stop listening to your hunger, you open up a can of worms. Then it is more likely that you won't listen to your "I'm satisfied" or "I'm comfortable cues," and you might start overeating.

Know your food triggers

Many of us have developed certain triggers (environmental or emotional) that contribute to habits of overeating. Figuring out what these triggers are for you is a first, important step toward squelching overeating. When your next food craving strikes (especially if you aren't physically hungry at the time), try to figure out what brought it on.

Sensory triggers: Things you see, smell, or taste that make you want to eat (television commercials, walking past a particular restaurant).

- _____
- _____
- _____

Verbal triggers: Things you hear that make you want to eat (someone talking about how great something tastes, someone telling you you've gained weight).

- _____
- _____
- _____

Emotional triggers: Your psychological state or feelings that increase your desire to eat (being anxious, depressed, happy, bored).

- _____
- _____
- _____

Other triggers:

Anything else that triggers cravings for certain foods when you aren't physically hungry.

- _____
- _____
- _____

Binge Eating Disorder

Binge Eating Disorder: eating larger amounts of food than most people would eat in a certain period of time (that is, two hours) with a sense of lack of control during these episodes.

Occurrence: It is estimated to occur in 20 to 50 percent of people who seek specialized obesity treatment.

Characteristics: Obese people with Binge Eating Disorder tend to be heavier, report greater psychological distress, and are more likely to have experienced a psychiatric illness than obese people without Binge Eating Disorder. They may have spent a great percentage of their lifetime on a diet and/or their weight may have fluctuated and cycled greatly over their lifetime.

Maximize your calorie burning

Should you eat fewer calories? You could, but that isn't very much fun. Your body needs more of various nutrients as you age anyway. If you eat less, you aren't likely to be getting more of these nutrients (such as calcium, vitamin D, antioxidants, vitamin B-12, zinc, and so on). And there are so many other health benefits to the following suggestions. You are truly better off burning more calories rather than eating a lot less. Here's how to burn more calories:

Exercising. Exercising, in general, helps increase the number of calories you burn in a day. Of course we know we burn the extra calories while we exercise, but some new evidence suggests we even burn extra calories after we exercise (possibly four to 12 hours after exercise). When you just begin to exercise regularly, you use mostly glucose (carbohydrate) as your main fuel during aerobic exercise. Once you get into a regular exercise program and your body becomes more fit, your body will start to burn more fat for the extra energy you need while you are exercising. Generally after exercising 20 minutes, the new exerciser is probably primarily burning fat for fuel. Go for at least 20 minutes of valuable fat-burning time, then, you want to strive for those aerobic workouts that go for at least 40 minutes.

Grazing is good!

Eating small frequent meals throughout the day and eating light at night, is the best way to spread your calories out metabolically speaking (and weight loss wise too). For more on this, check out Food Step to Freedom 1 in Chapter 3.

Build muscle to burn more calories. Muscle cells burn more calories at rest than fat cells do. How many calories are we talking about? About 70 percent of the calories you burn in a day are due to the metabolic activity of your lean body mass (muscle). If you want to build muscle tissue instead of fat tissue, exercise has to be part of your plan. For the best results use a combination of aerobic conditioning and strength training, especially during and after menopause.

Eat breakfast. Your metabolism (the rate at which the body burns calories) may slow down to conserve fuel. One of the biggest gaps in eating is night time, when we sleep. If you are one of those people who isn't hungry right when you wake up, drink a small glass of juice or milk, then pack some food to bring with you wherever you go. An hour or two later, when your hunger kicks in, you will be prepared.

Eat small, frequent meals through the day, and eat light at night. Each time you eat, you set your body's digestive process in motion. Each time you start it up, you burn calories. So the more frequently you eat, the more calories you burn just by digesting your food.

Burn more calories digesting high-carbohydrate whole foods. Your body uses more energy (burns more calories) to metabolize carbohydrates than it does to break down dietary fat. For example, if you eat 100 high-fat potato chips calories in excess of your calorie needs, about 97 of the 100 calories will probably end up as fat storage. But if you eat 100 higher carbohydrate calories as a baked potato, for example, 77 calories will probably be deposited as fat (because your body burned 23 calories to digest, convert, and store those mostly carbohydrate calories).

How to maintain your muscle mass

Muscle mass and muscle strength also tends to decline as you age, because you start losing more and more muscle fibers and nerves that stimulate them. But you enhance your muscle mass through strength training and regular exercise. In terms of diet, you should make sure you are getting enough protein, but not too much. In this case, more is not better. The only true way to *build* muscle is to *use* muscle.

Start strength training, like, yesterday!

Anyone can start boosting their muscle mass by doing appropriate strength-training exercises two to three times a week. You may have heard of these other terms for strength training: resistance training, weight training, and isotonics. Strength-training exercises usually involve activities that you repeat eight to 12 times in a row while standing or sitting in one place. The exercises pull a muscle (or set of muscles) to exhaustion. This encourages the muscle to grow and improve its tone. Strength training can be done two to three times a week for 30 to 40 minutes each session. Here are four great reasons to start strength training now!

1. Strength training builds muscle mass. Because muscle mass requires *more* calories to sustain itself than body fat, strength training helps raise your metabolic rate.

2. Strength training increases bone density, so it also helps reduce the risk of osteoporosis.

3. The more muscle you have, the less insulin is required to get sugar from the blood to body tissues. Strength training helps reduce your risk of developing diabetes in your later years.

4. Strength training can ease the pain of osteoarthritis and may even ease the pain of rheumatoid arthritis.

Q: So why are Americans getting heavier?

Those darn weight tables keep coming out. More diet books keep getting published. New drugs, herbal and otherwise, keep coming on the market. Jenny Craig, Weight Watchers, Slim Fast, and other billion-dollar dieting giants have been waging war against weight gain for decades now! Never before have more reduced-fat and reduced sugar foods been available. And yet, we are only getting heavier. What's going on? Getting back to the basics of weight control sheds some light on this rather sore subject.

One of the first questions related to weight control is: Do the "calories in" equal the "calories out"? That's because the net effect of excess calories (more than the body needs), even in the form of carbohydrates or protein, is going to increase the amount of fat put into storage (body fat). We know that most Americans haven't exactly been increasing their "calories out" side of the equation.

Due to a combination of modern life factors (TV, long commutes, computers, and so on), Americans have become more sedentary.

What about the "calories in" portion? True, the average person ate less fat as a percentage of total calories during the National Center for Health Statistics survey period (from 36 to 34 percent)—but the amount of daily calories went up an average of 231 calories in 1990 compared to 1976. Now we're getting to the million-dollar question: Why would Americans suddenly increase their total daily calories at a time when the country has never been more obsessed with dieting and more concerned about healthy eating.

Ironically, some researchers think it is exactly this overemphasis on fat-free foods that has contributed to the rampant weight gain. Perhaps this wave has fed the belief that if a food has little or no fat, you can have as much as you want without gaining weight. Perhaps when people eat mediocre-tasting fat-free foods, it leaves them feeling unsatisfied, so they eat more of the fat-free products or end of eating something else in the hopes of satisfying their hunger or food craving. Maybe since a large chunk of the American population is actively dieting at any one time, they continue to ride the unfortunate weight roller coaster of strict dieting and obsession, over and over again.

I'm eating healthy and exercising, so why am I not losing weight?

If you are exercising regularly and strength training as well, you are probably adding muscle weight while decreasing some body fat. Remember, muscle weighs more than body fat. Your weight could very well stay the same even though you are building muscle and losing body fat. Keep in mind—you are healthier for it.

You could also take a look at portion sizes. It is possible, even if you are choosing healthful foods, that the portions may be too large for your caloric needs. If you keep this up, your won't see any actual lost "pounds." Or, if you eat out often, you may be eating more calories or fat grams than you realize.

The dieting craze isn't helping

Experience shows that each time you lose weight you tend to gain it back and then some. And each time you do this you make it that much more difficult to lose the weight the next time you try. We have definitely been dieting (it's a billion dollar a year industry) and we are definitely gaining it back and then some, so this could be one big reason why we are getting heavier.

It comes down to calories?

With all the new fat-free cookies and light products out there—how did this weight surplus happen? We are now in a culture where food is fast. Many of us eat out more than we eat in. Sweets are all around us. And soda is the number-one source of added sugars.

As a nation, we have become very aware of low-fat diets, and because of that we have been eating more fat-free and low-fat products. But what we don't realize is, in many of these products, it's the sugar that is being substituted for the fat—with the calories staying pretty much the same. So we have really been trading fat for sugar. If the taste is only "alright" or if we are in the mindset that we can eat more because it's "fat-free," then we are actually eating more (and getting more calories) with some of the products.

Surveys have shown that we are eating fewer percent calories from fat than 15 to 20 years ago, but they are also showing that we are eating *more calories* and more added sugars. We are actually eating 300 more calories a day when you compare data between 1975 and 1995. Not good, especially when you factor in we are less active (burning fewer calories) than we were back then.

Reducing dietary fat alone, without reducing calories, is not going to encourage weight loss. But if you reduce fat along with reducing carbohydrates, calories will decrease and weight loss will be possible.

If we ate more fruits, vegetables, beans, and whole grains, we would be eating fewer calories per a certain volume of food compared to the type of eating style filled with high-fat meat, processed and sweet food fare.

If we are eating less fat and we are only getting fatter, then should we eat more fat to lose weight?

First of all, that's not really true, we aren't really eating less fat. Although Americans consume fewer "percent calories from fat" the actual number of grams that we take in has actually increased from 81 to 83 grams a day. How can the percent calories from fat decrease if we are eating 2 grams more fat per day? Because we have been eating *more calories* per day. So what's the big deal between eating 81 and 83 grams of fat a day, you ask?

This computes out to an extra:

- 18 extra fat calories a day.
- 126 extra fat calories a week.
- 540 extra fat calories a month.
- 6,500 extra fat calories a year.

An important piece of the puzzle—exercise

Working on our "calories out" side of the weight loss equation is a must—along with our food choices and amounts (the "calories in" portion of the equation). There are a few ways to increase our calories out—or the amount of calories we burn or use up as fuel. Exercise plays an important role in the first two ways.

1. We can move our body more and exercise, which requires calories.
2. We can increase our muscle in our body, which increases our metabolic rate.

3. We can adjust our food choices to maximize calorie burning due to digestion.

How to start exercising— even if you are a couch potato

The bottom line is that physical activity can make the difference between losing weight and not losing weight. And if that isn't enough to get you off the couch, regular exercise has been shown to lower high triglyceride levels in the blood and lower high blood pressure after only 10 weeks. The risk of heart attack also decreases with regular exercise.

Exercise has psychological benefits too—it simply makes you feel better. It encourages better sleep, gives you more energy throughout the day, helps you feel better about your body even if pounds haven't been lost, and it also helps reduce depression and stress.

Of the above benefits though, helping us trim extra fat around the middle and helping reduce stress are the two benefits most likely to help your acid reflux symptoms.

I can go over and over all the various benefits of exercise, and I can even hold your hand and follow you around for a month helping you get in the habit of exercising. But sooner or later it is all going to come back to one person—you. Ultimately you have to take responsibility for your exercise habits.

The first step is to commit to trying "exercise" for one month, remembering to start slowly. At the end of one month you should hopefully have experienced many of the psychological and physiological benefits of exercise, and you will be adequately "hooked." So let's look at how to get started:

- Visit your doctor and make sure you can proceed with your plans to start exercising.
- Don't make it a big weight-loss contest—focus on health and gaining better control of your blood sugar.

- It has to be fun or you are definitely not going to stick with it.

- Next, find out what your exercise preferences and needs are and try to consider them when making your exercise plans.

- Do you like exercising indoors or outdoors?

- Do you like to exercise alone, with a partner, or with a group?

- Do you like the gym atmosphere?

- At what time of day would you be most likely to stick to exercising?

- Do you have any physical limitations that need to be considered? If you have joint limitations, for example, water aerobics or swimming can actually be a great starting place.

- What do you like to do? Even if your answer is watching television or talking, they can be worked into your exercise program. If you like to talk, walking with a partner might be the ticket. If you like to watch television, then home exercise equipment that you can use in the comfort of your family room or bedroom might be your most practical option.

Read this before you start exercising if you have acid reflux

Don't exercise, particularly by doing activities that involve bending or running, soon after eating. When you bend over or jump around with a somewhat full stomach, your stomach is bending and jumping too—encouraging stomach acid to reflux into the lower esophagus. Find out when your body is most comfortable exercising. For me it's either after work but before dinner, or it's several hours after dinner but before bed. (I like to ride my stationary bike while I watch some of my favorite evening TV shows.) For others it might be first thing in the morning.

Give it two hours! If you find your heartburn seems to get worse after exercise, try waiting at least two hours after a meal before you exercise and see if that helps.

Every little bit helps

Even if you can't imagine exercising 30 minutes or more in one sitting, split it up into three 10-minute mini-workouts. Ten minutes of activity here and there does add up to health benefits for your body. Any way that you can increase your activity throughout your day will help your cause.

Strength training gives you more than strength

The more muscle you have, the more calories and fat you burn—even sitting at the computer. That's because the more muscle you have, the higher your metabolic rate (the amount of calories your body burns just maintaining itself). So how do we make more muscle? The only way to build muscle is to use muscle. A great way to work your muscles directly is by strength training or resistance training.

But before you buy dumbbells, keep these things in mind:

- Consult your doctor and a strength-training instructor. The exercises must be done properly to prevent injury to build muscle strength.
- Do exercises in front of a mirror at first, to be sure your form matches the instructor (especially if you are working from a strength-training video).
- Start off strengthening the largest muscles in your body (muscles in the legs, back, and chest). You'll get the biggest metabolic bang for your buck this way.

- Start with whatever weight you feel comfortable lifting, but generally, you want to lift a weight that's heavy enough to make you feel fatigued after nine or so repititions. Starting out with overly heavy weights can lead to injuries.

- According to the American College of Sports Medicine, a single set of six to 12 repetitions is a great place to start. For beginners, single sets are just as effective as multiple sets.

Q: Quick weight loss—what are you really losing?

You know those books and magazine articles claiming you can "lose five pounds in five days"? You can only be losing mostly water if you lose five pounds in five days. Let me show you what you are really losing in those first few days.

Days 1–3 of a quick weight loss diet

- 75 percent of the weight loss is water.
- 20 percent of the weight loss is fat.
- 5 percent of the weight loss is protein.

Days 11–13

- 69 percent of the weight loss is fat.
- 9 percent of the weight loss is water.
- 12 percent of the weight loss is protein.

Days 21–24

- 85 percent of the weight loss is fat.
- 15 percent of the weight loss is protein.
- 0 percent of the weight loss is water.

Q: So what can we do?

- **Stop dieting!** We know it doesn't work. We know it actually works against you. If you think back to your past experiences, you will know this to be true—if you are being honest with yourself.

- **Eat when you're hungry and stop when you are comfortable.** When you "diet" you force yourself not to listen to your natural hunger cues. When you do this, you also tend *not* to listen to your "comfortable" cues and overeat at times. In order to stop overeating, you need to stop dieting and start listening to when your body truly is comfortable.

- **Start exercising!** Exercising helps your body in so many ways. It is one of the fastest ways to increase your "calories out" side of the equation. (See page 89 for tips on how to start exercising—even if you're a couch potato.)

- **Eat a high fiber (lower fat) diet**…that celebrates whole foods instead of fast or processed foods.

Chapter 5

How to Have a Heartburn-Free Holiday

Ask any heartburn sufferer if there is a time of year when they tend to be particularly uncomfortable and most will tell you "the holiday season." For many, it's a given. If it's the holidays, then get ready for heartburn.

That's because this is the no-holds-barred time of year when we break any food rules we may have had during the year. We are celebrating the season, and with all the festivities, overindulgence is sure to follow—along with the worst acid reflux you've ever known. This is the last thing you want or need during this time of year. Even the stress of the holidays can add to the acid reflux risk.

Think about how we eat during the holiday season. We do exactly the opposite of the 10 Food Steps to Freedom:

- We indulge in high-fat foods and foods we don't normally have, such as rich sauces and gravies, rich desserts, eggnog, marbled meats, and creamy cheeses.
- We literally "feast" at our holiday feasts—eating large amounts of food at one sitting.
- We often eat these extra large meals in the evening, just a few hours before we turn in for the night.

- Wine and spiked eggnog is flowing, alcohol is another given.

- And I would go so far as to say that tight clothing is a given too. (Tight clothing puts pressure on the stomach, which can help push stomach contents up into the esophagus.)

So, to help you have a heartburn-free holiday, I've put together some quick tips and some party recipes to shed some "light" on holiday eating. Of course if you are going to use the holiday recipes, there's a little catch. (Isn't there always?) You, or someone you love, will have to cook at least part of the holiday meal. But don't panic, these recipes are not only light in fat and calories, but they're light on time and effort too. This chapter hopefully covers the bases with recipes for everything from appetizers to favorite holiday side dishes to delectable desserts.

Q. So what can I do to avoid heartburn during the holidays?

Stuffing ourselves with food we don't eat but once a year, eating lots of rich and fatty food, and eating and drinking late into the night...that's what inevitably happens during the holidays. All of this is loads of fun until the heartburn hits with a vengeance. Here are 11 tips to get you through the holidays—hopefully heartburn free.

11 tips toward a heartburn-free holiday

1. Don't lie down on a full stomach. Stop eating and drinking around 7 p.m., then turn in around 11 p.m., once the stomach contents have mostly left the stomach.

2. Try to avoid eating large amounts of the foods that tend to relax the lower esophageal sphincter or encourage heartburn in other ways (onions, chocolate, fatty foods, citrus fruits, tomato juice, carbonated drinks, coffee, caffeinated tea, caffeinated soda, and alcoholic drinks). The calcium in milk may increase stomach acid secretion, so you might tolerate smaller amounts of milk, but have trouble with larger portions.

3. Another reason to avoid eating a lot of high-fat foods is that the higher the fat in your meal, the longer it will linger in your stomach before going on to the small intestine. This means the stomach will be full of potentially troubling foodstuffs longer!

4. Avoid eating foods that can directly irritate an already inflamed esophagus (citrus juices, citrus fruit and tomato products, pepper and chili pepper).

5. Avoid drinking beverages, particularly before bedtime, which can encourage heartburn (soft drinks, coffee, citrus juices, tomato juice, and alcohol). If you avoid soft drinks, coffee, and alcohol, what's left? Basically water, non-carbonated decaf beverages, and non-citrus fruit juices may be an option for some. If you decide to imbibe in soft drinks, coffee, or alcohol, at least try and keep it to a minimum—keep it to one precious cup.

6. Avoid bending over, doing any heavy lifting, or running after a big meal. This can increase pressure in the stomach and can aggravate heartburn.

7. Relax during the holidays—if you can. Emotional stress and anxiety can aggravate heartburn.

8. Keep portions to a minimum. As hard and impossible as this sounds, try not to eat those "eat till you explode" large meals. Passing up "seconds" will usually

do the trick. I know everything tastes so good, so bring some leftovers home and enjoy the whole dinner again—tomorrow.

9. Make better choices. When confronted with the typical party/holiday nibbles, know which ones are less likely to give you trouble (which is probably the ones lower in fat).

10. Offer to bring food to the party or holiday meal that you know you can eat without problems. You can bring low-fat (or low-spice) renditions of favorite party foods, if your system tends to have trouble with this. Make a lower fat dip using fat-free or light sour cream. Make a low-fat spread (such as crab or salmon) by using light cream cheese and cut out any added butter completely. And don't forget to eat slowly and enjoy it!

11. Especially throughout the holiday season, focus on including high-fiber foods (not on the avoid list) in every meal.

Thanksgiving menu ideas

What's Thanksgiving dinner without turkey and all the trimmings; heaps of fluffy, white potatoes doused in thick gravy; the scoops of moist and savory stuffing, sweet potatoes baked in a glaze of butter and brown sugar; and a hefty wedge of pumpkin pie?

No one here is trying to take away the traditional flavors of Thanksgiving, believe me. We have ways of making mashed potatoes, gravy, stuffing, sweet potatoes, and pie a few pounds lighter (in fat) without compromising taste and integrity. I've taken the liberty of developing lighter versions of some traditional Thanksgiving fixings. I hope they bring you comfort and enjoyment!

Lightened Thanksgiving recipes

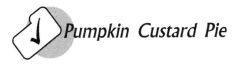 **Pumpkin Custard Pie**

Makes 12 servings.

- 1/3 cup sugar
- 1/3 cup brown sugar
- 3/4 tsp. ground cinnamon
- 1/2 tsp. ground nutmeg (replace with cinnamon, if this irritates your stomach)
- Pinch of ground cloves
- 1 1/2 cups canned pumpkin
- 1 tsp. vanilla extract
- 1 1/4 cups evaporated skim milk
- 1 Tbs. freshly grated orange peel
- 3 egg whites, lightly beaten
- 1/4 cup Meyers rum (or brandy). Orange juice can be substituted as well
- Single pie crust (see the high-fiber pie crust recipe in Chapter 6)

1. Preheat oven to 425 degrees.
2. In a mixing bowl, combine sugars, cinnamon, nutmeg, and cloves. Stir in pumpkin. Add vanilla, evaporated milk, orange peel, and egg whites. Beat with an electric mixer until smooth. Fold in rum.
3. Pour into a 9-inch unbaked pie crust and bake for 10 minutes. Reduce heat to 325 degrees and bake for 45 minutes or until knife inserted in the filling comes out clean. Let cool and refrigerate until served. Serve with light Cool Whip or a dollop of whipping cream if desired.

Per serving: 180 calories, 4.5 g protein, 27 g carbohydrate, 6 g fat, 1 mg cholesterol, 1 gram fiber, 145 mg sodium. Calories from fat: 30 percent.

Quick Sherry Cake (with Hot Buttered Sherry Glaze)

Makes 12 servings.

- Cooking spray
- 1 box Duncan Hines moist deluxe butter recipe golden cake mix (or similar)
- 1 package (4 serving size) instant vanilla pudding mix
- 1/2 tsp. ground nutmeg (replace with cinnamon if necessary)
- 1 large egg
- 1/2 cup egg substitute
- 3/4 cup cream sherry
- 2 Tbs. canola oil
- 1/2 cup and 2 Tbs. fat-free sour cream (light can be substituted)

  Glaze:
- 1/2 cup powdered sugar
- 1 Tbs. cream sherry
- 1 Tbs. melted butter

1. Preheat oven to 375 degrees (if using a metal or glass pan) or 350 degrees (if using a dark or coated pan—and add three to five minutes to baking time). Coat sides and bottom of a Bundt or tube pan with cooking spray.

2. Combine cake mix, pudding mix, nutmeg, egg, egg substitute, sherry, oil, and sour cream in large mixing bowl. Blend at low speed until moistened (about 30 seconds). Scrape sides of bowl.

3. Beat at medium speed for exactly three minutes. Pour batter in prepared pan and bake immediately (place in center of oven). Bake for about 33 to 35 minutes. Cake is done when toothpick inserted in center of cake comes out clean. Cool in pan on rack for 15 minutes.

4. While cake is cooling, blend glaze ingredients in 1 cup measuring cup. Poke holes in top of cake with fork. Drizzle glaze over the top of cake and enjoy!

Per serving: 313 calories, 6 g protein, 50 g carbohydrate, 7.5 g fat, 1.5 g saturated fat, 20 mg cholesterol, .6 g fiber, 267 mg sodium. Calories from fat: 22 percent.

Potatoes With Leeks and Gruyere

This is a super dish for a holiday dinner—it can even be assembled a day in advance—just bake it on the big day. It can even be baked, cooled, covered, and refrigerated the day before. Just rewarm, covered, in 350-degree oven for about 25 minutes.

Makes 12 servings.

- 1 Tbs. olive oil or canola oil
- 1 lb. leeks (white and pale green parts only), thinly sliced
- 8 oz. package of light cream cheese, room temperature
- 1 tsp. salt
- 1 tsp. ground black pepper
- 1/4 tsp. ground nutmeg (or cinnamon)
- 1 cup low-fat milk
- 1 large egg
- 1/2 cup egg substitute
- 2 lbs. frozen shredded hash browns, thawed somewhat

- 2 cups grated Gruyere cheese (about 8 oz.)
- 1 tsp. of parsley flakes or Italian herb blend, or fines herbs

1. Preheat oven to 350 degrees. Coat a 9 × 13-inch baking dish with canola cooking spray.

2. Add olive oil to large nonstick skillet over medium heat. Add leeks and sauté until tender (about eight minutes). Remove from heat and set aside.

3. Blend cream cheese, salt, pepper, and nutmeg in food processor mixer. Slowly add milk and eggs one at a time, if using a mixer and beat just until blended. (Otherwise dump both the milk and eggs in the food processor and pulse just until blended). Stir leeks, shredded potatoes, and Gruyere into milk mixture and pour into prepared baking dish. Sprinkle parsley flakes or herb blend over the top if desired.

4. Bake dish until cooked through and top is brown (about 50 to 60 minutes). Cool slightly and serve.

Per serving: 217 calories, 11.5 g protein, 24 g carbohydrate, 8.5 g fat, 4.5 g saturated fat, 41 mg cholesterol, 2 g fiber, 340 mg sodium. Calories from fat: 35 percent.

Sour Creamed Potatoes

Makes 6 servings.

- 3 medium russet potatoes
- 1 Tbs. butter, canola margarine, or canola diet margarine
- 5 Tbs. fat-free or light sour cream
- 3 Tbs. low-fat milk

- 1/2-1 tsp. minced or crushed garlic
- 2 to 3 green onions, white and part of green, chopped
- 1 1/2 Tbs. fresh parsley, chopped
- 6 Tbs. grated or shredded Parmesan cheese
- Add pepper to taste
- Reduced-fat grated sharp cheddar cheese (optional)

1. Microwave or bake potatoes until tender throughout. Cut lengthwise in half. Scoop out as much of the potato from the skin as possible and put in a mixing bowl. (Set potato skins aside.)

2. To potato, add butter, sour cream, milk, garlic, onions, parsley, and Parmesan cheese. Blend with a mixer until creamy. Add pepper if desired.

3. Spoon into potato skins and sprinkle the top with grated cheese if desired. Broil until lightly brown.

Per serving: 163 calories, 6 g protein, 27 g carbohydrates, 3.5 g fat, 5 mg cholesterol, 2.5 g fiber, 159 mg sodium. Calories from fat: 19 percent.

Creamy Green Bean Bake

Makes 6 servings.
- 4 cups lightly cooked French-style frozen green beans
- 10 3/4-oz. can condensed Healthy Request cream of mushroom soup (or similar)
- 1/2 cup fat-free or light sour cream
- 1 Tbs. diced pimento (optional)
- 1/4 cup canned chow mein fried noodles (in Asian food section of your supermarket)

1. Lightly cook frozen beans if you haven't already. Preheat oven to 350 degrees.

2. In a 1-quart casserole dish or 9 x 9-inch dish, combine condensed soup, sour cream, and pimento. Measure 4 cups of cooked green beans, add to dish, and stir.

3. Bake for 20 minutes or until bubbly. Sprinkle chow mein noodles over the top and bake five minutes more.

Per serving: 102 calories, 4 g protein, 16 g carbohydrate, 2 gram fat, 2 mg cholesterol, 3 g fiber, 337 mg sodium. Calories from fat: 20 percent.

O'Brien Potato Casserole

Makes 16 servings.

- 2 lbs. Ore-Ida Potatoes O'Brien (about 8 cups)
- 2 cups fat-free or light sour cream
- 6 green onions, white and part of green, finely chopped
- 10 3/4-oz. can Healthy Request condensed cream of mushroom soup (or similar)
- 1/2 cup low-fat milk
- 2 Tbs. butter sprinkles (such as Molly McButter)
- 8 oz. shredded reduced-fat sharp cheddar cheese
- 1/2 tsp. salt
- 1/2 tsp. pepper
- 2 oz. Reduced-fat Ruffles potato chips, crushed (optional)

1. Preheat oven to 325 degrees. Coat a 13 × 9-inch baking pan with canola cooking spray.

2. Thaw potatoes and combine with all ingredients except the potato chips. Spread into prepared pan and top with crushed chips if desired. Bake for about 30 minutes.

Per serving: 115 calories, 7 g protein, 14.5 g carbohydrate, 3 g fat, 1 g fiber, 10 mg cholesterol, 308 mg sodium. Calories from fat: 26 percent.

Apple Sweet Potato Bake

Makes 6 servings.
- Canola cooking spray
- 5 cups thinly sliced sweet potatoes (or yams)
- 2 cups thinly sliced apples
- 1/4 cup plus 2 Tbs. brown sugar, packed
- 2 Tbs. maple syrup
- 1/2 tsp. ground cinnamon
- 1/2 cup apple juice
- 4 Tbs. chopped walnuts

1. Preheat oven to 350 degrees. Coat a 9 × 9-inch baking dish with canola cooking spray.

2. In a large bowl, toss the first three ingredients together. Spoon into the prepared baking dish.

3. In a small bowl, blend syrup with cinnamon. Add apple juice and stir to blend. Pour evenly over sweet potato mixture. Sprinkle walnuts over the top. Cover with foil and bake for 30 minutes.

4. Remove foil and bake about 20 minutes longer or until apple and sweet potatoes are cooked throughout.

Per serving: 193 calories, 2.5 g protein, 38.5 g carbohydrate, 3 g fat, 0 mg cholesterol, 3.5 g fiber, 14 mg sodium. Calories from fat: 15 percent.

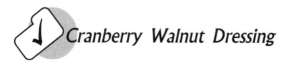

Cranberry Walnut Dressing

Eliminate the onions if they are one of your heartburn trigger foods.

Makes about 16 (1 cup each) servings.

- 1 1/2 cups finely sliced celery hearts
- 1 1/2 cups chopped onion (1 large onion)
- 3 Tbs. butter or canola margarine
- 1 cup reduced sodium chicken broth (liquid)
- 16 oz. can whole berry cranberry sauce
- 4 tsp. or cubes of low-sodium chicken broth (powder)
- 2 cups reduced sodium chicken broth (liquid)
- 3/4 tsp. ground sage
- 1 tsp. thyme
- 1/2 tsp. ground pepper
- 14 oz. (about 8 cups) herb-seasoned bread cubes for stuffing
- 2/3 cup walnuts, toasted for 1 minute under broiler to lightly brown

1. In a Dutch oven or stock pot, simmer celery and onion in the butter and 1 cup chicken broth until tender.

2. While onion and celery mixture is simmering, in a small saucepan mix cranberry sauce with the 4 tsp. of chicken broth powder over low heat until broth powder dissolves.

3. Add seasonings and 2 cups chicken broth to celery-onion mixture. Add bread cubes and stir until evenly moistened. Drizzle cranberry mixture over the top of the bread mixture and sprinkle walnuts over cranberry mixture. Stir to mix evenly. Cover and let sit on warm setting of stove for about 20 minutes, stirring occasionally.

Per serving: 200 calories, 4.5 g protein, 32.5 g carbohydrate, 5.8 g fat, 6 mg cholesterol, 415 mg sodium. Calories from fat: 26 percent.

Happy hour hints—party on!

You walk in and look around. As you are greeted with an eggnog, you try to remember if this is your third or fourth holiday party this week. You grab a handful of those cute as can be Christmas M&Ms on your way to talk with a friend. While talking, you nibble on a couple handfuls of chips and dip and crackers and cheese. Later, when champagne is passed around, you try pieces of English toffee and fudge sitting on the coffee table, on top of several toothpicks of fancy sausage that you had somewhere between the chocolate and the champagne. By the time you walk out of the party, you have racked up a total of around 2,200 calories, most of which are from fat.

I'm not suggesting we all roam around our holiday parties drinking water and chewing on celery sticks. But we can save ourselves from post-party heartburn by partying with a little extra food wisdom. Start by taking the 11 Tips Toward A Heartburn-Free Holiday to heart. Then check out some of these heartburn-friendly appetizer recipes.

Salmon Spread

Makes about 2 cups of spread.

- 7 1/2 oz. of freshly cooked salmon or smoked salmon
- 1/2 cup light cream cheese
- 1/4 cup part-skim or low-fat ricotta cheese
- 1/3 cup (heaped) jicama or canned water chestnuts (well drained), finely chopped
- 1/4 cup white onion, finely chopped (optional)
- 1 Tbs. parsley flakes
- 1/2 tsp. black pepper
- 1 loaf multi-grain French bread, cut into 16 slices

1. Mix all ingredients (except bread), very briefly, in food processor. Stir the mixture around, scraping sides of food processor bowl, and briefly blend again. Keep well chilled (you can make this a day before you need it).

2. Spread 1 Tbs. of spread on each 1/2 slice of bread.

Per 1/2 slice of bread: 59 calories, 3.5 g protein, 8 g carbohydrate, 1.5 g fat, .5 g saturated fat, 5 mg cholesterol, 2 g fiber, 105 mg sodium. Calories from fat: 22 percent.

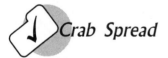

Crab Spread

Makes about 2 cups of spread.

- 6 oz. fresh crab, shredded
- 1/2 cup light cream cheese, at room temperature
- 1/4 cup plain yogurt
- 1 Tbs. onion flakes (optional)
- 1 Tbs. parsley flakes

- 1/2 tsp. black pepper
- 1/8 tsp. salt
- 1/3 cup chopped water chestnuts or jicama
- Lowfat and whole wheat crackers (or similar)

1. Mix crab, cream cheese, yogurt, and seasonings together in mixer on low speed. Stir in water chestnuts or jicama.

2. Serve with whole grain crackers.

Per 1/8 cup of spread: 114 calories, 10 g protein, 4 g carbohydrate, 6.5 g fat, 3.5 g saturated fat, 36 mg cholesterol, 2 g fiber, 311 mg sodium. Calories from fat: 51 percent.

Spinach Dip (in Sourdough Round)

Makes 12 appetizer servings.

- 1 round multigrain sourdough bread loaf (about 24 oz.)
- 1/3 cup real mayonnaise (substitute 2/3 cup light mayonnaise and decrease fat-free sour cream to 1 1/3 cup if desired)
- 1 2/3 cup fat-free or light sour cream
- 5 oz. can sliced water chestnuts, drained and chopped
- 5 green onions, white and part of green, chopped (optional)
- 1 package leek, onion, or vegetable soup mix (such as Knorr Soup Mix)
- 10 oz. box frozen chopped spinach; thaw and squeeze out excess water

1. Cut out top and center portion of sourdough round to make a bowl for the spinach dip. Cut the remaining bread into cubes for dipping.

2. In medium-sized bowl, blend mayonnaise and sour cream with soup mix powder. Stir in water chestnuts, onions if tolerated, and well-drained spinach.

3. Spread into sourdough bowl. Serve with bread cubes.

Per serving: 253 calories, 8 g protein, 39.5 g carbohydrate, 6.5 g fat, 1 g saturated fat, 4 mg cholesterol, 5 g fiber, 500 mg sodium. Calories from fat: 24 percent.

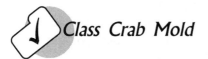

Class Crab Mold

Makes 16 spread servings.

- 8 oz. crab meat (fresh, frozen, or canned, drained well and patted dry)
- 1 can Campbell's Healthy Request Cream of Mushroom Soup (or similar), concentrated
- 1 envelope Knox plain, unflavored gelatin
- 8 oz. light cream cheese
- 1/4 cup real mayonnaise (substitute light mayonnaise if desired)
- 3/4 cup fat-free or light sour cream
- 1/2 cup chopped green onions (if tolerated)
- 1 cup finely chopped celery

  Serving suggestion: serve with thinly sliced multigrain French or sourdough baguette, multigrain or wheat low-fat crackers.

1. Heat concentrated cream of mushroom soup in medium saucepan over medium low heat. Add gelatin and cream cheese and let it come to a gentle boil. Let boil, stirring frequently, until cream cheese melts and gelatin dissolves. Remove from heat.

2. Stir in mayonnaise, sour cream, crab, green onions if tolerated, and celery. Spread into 1 quart mold or larger, and refrigerate until set.

Per serving (spread only): 84 calories, 6 g protein, 4 g carbohydrate, 5 g fat, 1.5 g saturated fat, 21 mg cholesterol, .2 g fiber, 258 mg sodium. Calories from fat: 54 percent.

Light and High-Fiber Cloverleaf Rolls

We cut almost a stick of butter from this recipe, lowered the fat from milk, decreased the salt, eliminated the egg yolk, and used more than half whole wheat flour!

Makes 16 rolls.

- 1 cup and 3 Tbs. lowfat milk, make warm to the touch by heating briefly in the microwave
- 3 Tbs. granulated sugar
- 3 Tbs. canola oil
- 1/4 cup fat free sour cream
- Pinch or two of freshly ground nutmeg (optional)
- 2 cups whole-wheat flour
- 1 3/4 cups unbleached white flour
- 1 teaspoon salt
- 1 package (.25 ounce) or 2 1/2 teaspoons rapid rise or bread machine yeast
- Canola cooking spray

1. Set bread machine to "dough" cycle and add the ingredients into the bread machine pan in the order listed or follow the instructions of your bread machine manufacturer if different from the following:

2. Add the milk. Sugar, canola oil, sour cream, and nutmeg into the pan. Then add the whole-wheat flour and the white flour. Pour the salt into one corner of the pan and make a well in the center of the flour that's in the pan. Pour the yeast into the well.

3. Press "START" and the dough cycle should take about 1 hour and 40 minutes. Once that is complete, place dough on a lightly flour sheet of wax paper and lightly cover the ball of dough with the flour.

4. Coat the inside of 16 muffin cups with canola cooking spray and begin preheating the oven to 400-degrees with the rack in the middle position.

5. Cut the big ball of dough into four equal pieces. Then take one of the pieces and cut it into four more pieces (each of these pieces is equivalent to one roll). Take one of the roll pieces and cut it into three equal parts. Gently roll each part and place all three in one of the prepared muffin cups. Continue with the remaining three pieces (filling a total of four muffin cups).

6. Repeat with remaining dough to fill all 16-muffin cups. Spray the tops with canola cooking spray. Place muffin tins on or near the preheating oven (or anywhere fairly warm). Let rise, loosely covered with a thin kitchen towel until almost doubled in size (about 40 minutes). Bake until golden (15 to 20 minutes). Enjoy!

Per Roll: 143 calories, 4.5 g protein, 25 g carbohydrate, 3 g fat, .4 g saturated fat, 1.6 g monounsaturated fat, 1 g polyunsaturated fat, 1 mg cholesterol, 2.5 g fiber, 146 mg sodium. Calories from fat: 19 percent

High-Fiber Canola Oil Pie Crust

Makes 1, 9-inch deep dish single pie crust

- 3/4 cup whole wheat pastry flour (or regular whole wheat flour)
- 3/4 cup unbleached white flour
- 3/4 teaspoon salt
- 1 Tbs. light pancake syrup
- 5 Tbs. canola oil
- 3 Tbs. lowfat buttermilk

1. Add flours and salt to medium size bowl and blend well with electric mixer (on low)

2. Add the pancake syrup and canola oil to mixing bowl and beat on low speed until the mixture looks blended and crumbly. Pour in the buttermilk and mix on low speed just until the dough is moist and holds together well (about 15 seconds). Stir in a teaspoon or two more buttermilk if the dough seems a little too dry.

3. Using your hands, press dough evenly into your deep-dish pie plate. If the dough is a little thicker around the pie plate rim, you can pinch the dough into scallops or make the rim double thickness and press it with a fork around the circle, as desired.

4. Proceed with your recipe for baking. If you need a prebaked pie crust, preheat the oven to 375-degrees, poke the crust several times with a fork, and bake for about 20 minutes.

Per serving (if 12 servings): 111 calories, 2 g protein, 12 g carbohydrate, 6 g fat (.5 g saturated fat, 3.5 g monounsaturated fat, 1.8 g polyunsaturated fat), 0 mg cholesterol, 1 g fiber, 151 mg sodium. Calories from fat: 48 percent.

Fry Light Parsnip Pancakes

Makes 10 pancakes.

- 1 large egg (higher omega-3 if available)
- 1/4 cup egg substitute
- 2 Tbs. unbleached white flour
- 3 Tbs. fat-free half-and-half or low-fat milk
- 1/2 teaspoon black pepper
- 1/4 to 1/2 teaspoon salt
- 4 cups shredded (grated) parsnip
- 1 cup finely chopped carrot (you can grate the carrot then finely chop)
- 1/3 cup finely chopped scallions or green onions (white and part of green)
- 2 Tbs. canola oil

1. Add egg, egg substitute, and flour to a large mixing bowl and whisk until smooth. Whisk in the half-and-half or low-fat milk, pepper, and salt.

2. Add the parsnip, carrot, and scallions to the mixing bowl with egg mixture to toss together to blend well.

3. Start heating a large, nonstick frying pan over medium-high heat. Add 1 tablespoon of the canola oil and when it is nice and hot and covers the bottom of the frying pan evenly, use a 1/2-cup measure to form five pancakes (a scant 1/2-cup of batter each). Spray the tops of the pancakes with cooking spray if desired.

4. When underside of the pancakes is golden brown (about two minutes), flip pancakes over to lightly brown other side (about two minutes). Remove pancakes to serving plate.

5. Repeat steps 3 and 4 with remaining oil and pan-cake batter.

Per pancake: 83 calories, 3 g protein, 11 g carbohydrate, 3.5 g fat, .4 g saturated fat, 1.9 g monounsaturated fat, .9 g polyunsaturated fat, 26 mg cholesterol, 3 g fiber, 135 mg sodium (if 1/2 teaspoon salt) and 89 mg sodium (if 1/4 teaspoon salt). Calories from fat: 38 percent.

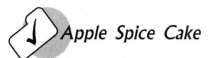

Apple Spice Cake

Makes 16 servings.

- 1 1/2 cups whole-wheat flour
- 1 1/2 cups unbleached white flour
- 1 Tbs. ground cinnamon
- 1 teaspoon baking soda
- 1 teaspoon salt
- 1 cup low-fat buttermilk
- 1/3 cup canola oil
- 1 1/2 cups granulated sugar
- 2 large eggs (high-omega-3 if available)
- 1/4 cup egg substitute or 2 egg whites
- 1 teaspoon vanilla extract
- 3 cups chopped apples—cored and sliced apples cut into 1/2-inch pieces (about 14 ounces of packaged sliced apples can be used)
- 3/4 cup coarsely chopped nuts—such as pecans or walnuts (optional)

1. Preheat oven to 350-degrees. Coat a 12-cup Bundt pan or tube pan with canola cooking spray; set aside.

2. Add flours, cinnamon, baking soda, and salt to medium bowl or 8-cup measuring cup and whisk to blend well.

3. Add buttermilk, canola oil, sugar, eggs, egg substitute, and vanilla to a large mixing bowl and with the paddle attachment, beat together on medium-high speed until smooth (about two minutes).

4. On low speed, slowly add in dry ingredients, mixing just until blended. Stir in chopped apples and nuts if desired. Pour into the prepared pan and bake until cake tester inserted in the cake comes out clean (about 1 hour and 15 minutes). Remove from oven and let the cake cool for 10 minutes then invert the cake onto a serving plate and remove the pan to help the cake cool completely.

Per serving: 225 calories, 4.5 g protein, 40 g carbohydrate, 5.5 g fat, .7 g saturated fat, 3 g monounsaturated fat, 1.6 g polyunsaturated fat, 27 mg cholesterol, 2.5 g fiber, 258 mg sodium. Calories from fat: 22 percent.

A holiday bonus for you!

With these "light" renditions of favorite holiday foods eaten in reasonable amounts, there is no acid reflux reason why we all can't enjoy holiday foods once a month instead of just once a year!

6 easy ways to reduce the richness in holiday foods

1. Most pumpkin pie recipes call for at least 1 cup of cream or evaporated whole milk and two eggs. Using evaporated skim and three egg whites will cut off about 300 calories and 30 to 38 grams of fat.

2. Buying brown and serve (bread) type rolls instead of the higher fat crescent rolls will cut out about 1,100 extra calories and about 100 grams of fat per dozen.

3. Using light cream cheese instead of regular cream cheese in your holiday dips, spreads, and cheesecakes will cut off about 16 grams of fat per cup of cream cheese.

4. Using a great-tasting fat-free sour cream (I recommend "Naturally Yours" brand in the black and white cow hide container) for your dips, spreads, and potato dishes will cut off about 320 calories and about 35 grams of fat per cup of sour cream.

5. Using reduced-fat cheese in your cheese logs, appetizers, and side dishes will cut off 36 grams of fat and 320 calories for every 8 ounces.

6. Making your dips and side dishes and appetizers with a mixture of real mayonnaise and fat-free sour cream. (For every cup of mayo, blend 1/4 cup mayo with 3/4 of fat-free sour cream.) This mix will cut out more than 1,000 calories and 132 grams of fat per cup of mayonnaise.

Chapter 6

Recipes You Can't Live Without

What types of recipes would be helpful in a book about acid reflux? Tums Tacos or Pepcid AC Cookies? No, take another gander at The 10 Food Steps to Freedom (Chapter 3) and a few patterns emerge.

I've come up with some no tomato options to our top tomato dishes (and eliminated the garlic and onion too, when possible). Please forgive me, but I couldn't come up with a no-tomato way of making spaghetti. I guess you could use a type of gravy instead of marinara sauce, but then that would be beef stroganoff, wouldn't it? I've even looked at 10 popular fatty foods and lightened them up so that you can eat fried chicken again!

Why is it so important to lighten up some of America's most fatty foods? (Other than the fact that food fat delays the emptying of the stomach into the small intestine, helps relax or weaken the esophageal sphincter valve, and a high-fat diet encourages weight gain.) When do people tend to have the most trouble with acid reflux? When they eat out. What have studies shown happens when people eat out? They eat a higher amount of fat (not to mention cholesterol and sodium too). So I looked at some of the favorite foods people eat when they eat breakfast out:

- eggs
- pancakes

I also looked at some of the favorite foods people eat when they eat lunch or dinner out:

- lettuce salads
- French fries
- mashed potatoes
- coleslaw
- pizza
- pasta
- chocolate chip cookies

I included lower-fat versions of as many of the previous items as I possibly could. If you enjoy these items enough to order them when you are out at the mall or in a restaurant, then you are bound to enjoy and appreciate these same foods when they are made lighter at home.

In the following recipes, just to keep the bases covered, obviously I've tried to honor the 10 Food Steps to Freedom whenever possible. Keep in mind everyone is going to be a little different. Some people have to eat spicy foods or high-tomato recipes with caution, while others find the greasy, fatty foods particularly problematic. Hopefully, no matter which food step to freedom you find gives the most relief, there will be a handful of recipes in this chapter that will help, not hurt, your heartburn.

No-tomato renditions for top tomato dishes

No-Tomato Lasagna (Creamy Pesto Lasagna)

Make up a batch of white sauce (page 138) and you're ready to throw this recipe together.

Makes 12 servings.

- 12 oz. (3/4 lb.) super lean ground beef (or ground sirloin)
- 1/3 cup (2.5 oz.) pesto (I use Armanino Pesto in the frozen food section)
- 1/2 cup beef broth
- 2 cups grated zucchini
- 1 1/2 cup part-skim ricotta cheese
- 2/3 cup chopped green onions (if tolerated)
- 12 oz. (dry weight) wide lasagna noodles (higher fiber)
- 2 cups low-fat white sauce *(see following recipe)*
- 6 oz. grated part-skim mozzarella cheese (1 1/2 cups)

1. Preheat oven to 375 degrees. Cook noodles in a large pot of boiling water until just tender (follow cooking directions on package). Drain well.

2. While boiling noodles, in nonstick frying pan coated with canola cooking spray, brown ground beef, breaking into small pieces with spatula as it cooks. Add browned beef to large bowl along with pesto, broth, and zucchini. Toss to blend well.

3. In a separate bowl, mix the ricotta with green onions.

4. To assemble lasagna:
   - Spread 1 cup of white sauce on bottom of 9 × 13-inch baking pan.

- Add three strips of lasagna noodles.
- Spread half of the beef mixture on top.
- Lay three strips of lasagna over the beef.
- Spread the ricotta cheese mixture on top.
- Add three strips of lasagna.
- Spread the remaining beef mixture on top of this.
- Add three strips of lasagna.
- Spread the very top with remaining white sauce.
- Sprinkle with the grated mozzarella.

Per serving: 318 calories, 19.5 g protein, 27 g carbohydrate, 14.5 g fat, 7 g saturated fat, 41 mg cholesterol, 5 g fiber (could be more depending on the noodle used), 316 mg sodium. Calories from fat: 40 percent.

Easy Low-Fat Alfredo Sauce

This is a sauce recipe for the Creamy Pesto Lasagna recipe, but it is a great entrée in it's own right. Just toss the sauce with roasted chicken breast strips, cooked prawns, or crumbled turkey bacon, and drizzle over cooked noodles, and you've got a marvelous variation of fettuccine alfredo!

Makes about 2 cups.

- 1/4 cup light cream cheese
- 1 1/4 cup low-fat or whole milk, divided
- 1 Tbs. Wondra quick-mixing flour
- 2 Tbs. butter (canola margarine can also be used), divided use
- 1/2 cup shredded Parmesan cheese
- Add salt and freshly grated pepper to taste
- Add nutmeg to taste (or cinnamon if nutmeg bothers your stomach)

1. Combine cream cheese, 1/4 cup whole milk, and flour in a small mixing bowl or food processor. Beat or pulse until well blended. Slowly pour in remaining milk (1 cup) and beat until smooth.

2. Melt 2 Tbs. butter in large, thick nonstick frying pan or saucepan over medium heat. Add the milk mixture and continue to heat, stirring constantly, until the sauce is just the right thickness (about four minutes).

3. Stir in grated Parmesan cheese and add salt, pepper, and nutmeg to taste if desired.

Per serving: If each 1/3 cup of sauce is served with 1 cup of cooked fettuccine noodles. 333 calories, 13 g protein, 43.5 g carbohydrate, 11.5 g fat, 6 g saturated fat, 31 mg cholesterol, 2 g fiber, 250 mg sodium. Calories from fat: 31 percent.

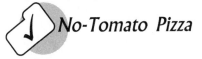 *No-Tomato Pizza*

Makes 2 servings (each serving is half a small pizza).

- 1 small packaged (ready-to-bake) whole grain pizza crust (5.5 oz.) such as Boboli brand or other (or use the high-fiber bread machine pizza crust recipe in this chapter)

- 2 Tbs. prepared pesto sauce (such as Armanino Farms in frozen food section) or quick ranch sauce (blend 1/8 cup fat-free or light sour cream with 1/2 tsp. Hidden Valley Ranch Dip powder from packet)

- 1/2 cup grated reduced-fat cheese (mozzarella, sharp cheddar, Jack, or a blend)

- 1/2 cup of toppings you know you can tolerate (such as a mixture of mushrooms, zucchini, lean ham, and pineapple, and so on)

1. Preheat oven to 400 degrees.
2. Place pizza crust on cookie sheet. Spread pesto or quick ranch sauce evenly over the crust. Top evenly with grated cheese and then the toppings of your choice.
3. Bake 8 to 12 minutes or until cheese is melted and crust lightly browned. Cut pizza in half.

Per serving (using pesto and zucchini and mushroom as the topping): 316 calories, 14.5 g protein, 36 g carbohydrate, 12 g fat, 4 g saturated fat, 18 mg cholesterol, 3 g fiber (this will be higher if the high-fiber pizza crust recipe is used), 580 mg sodium. Calories from fat: 35 percent.

10 Minute Spaghetti Carbonara (no egg yolk version)

I was trying to think of a way of making spaghetti without tomatoes and I thought it was a mission impossible, but then I remembered my recipe for spaghetti carbonara!

Makes 3 servings (2–4).

*   4 cups cooked whole wheat or whole wheat blend spaghetti noodles (until tender, but still a little firm), drained
*   1/4 cup egg substitute
*   1 Tbs. Wondra quick-mixing flour
*   1/2 cup plus 2 Tbs. double-strength chicken stock
*   1/4 cup dry white wine (champagne may also be used)
*   2 garlic cloves, minced—about 2 tsp. (if tolerated).
*   2 Tbs. butter and canola margarine
*   Salt and freshly ground pepper (optional)
*   4 slices turkey bacon, cooked carefully over medium-low heat and crumbled
*   2/3 cup freshly grated Parmesan cheese

1. Boil spaghetti noodles if you haven't already done so. In a small bowl, blend egg substitute with the Wondra flour; set aside.

2. In large nonstick skillet, combine the chicken broth, wine, garlic, and butter. Bring the mixture to a boil. Let boil gently for a minute or two. Turn off the heat. Season mixture with salt and pepper if desired.

3. Turn off heat. Add in the egg substitute mixture, stir well. Add the warm spaghetti noodles and toss well.

4. Stir in the crumbled turkey bacon and parmesan cheese and toss well.

Per serving: 396 calories, 18 g protein, 45 g carbohydrate, 14.5 g fat, 7.5 g saturated fat, 40 mg cholesterol, 6 g fiber, 860 mg sodium. Calories from fat: 35 percent.

Green Sauced Chicken Enchiladas

The green sauce in this recipe is made with tomatillos. Tomatillos are generally thought of as green Mexican tomatoes, but they are really botanically different from tomatoes. If you find you can tolerate tomatillos, then you have a simple solution to your favorite Mexican foods. Bottled salsa verde (made with tomatillos) can be used as salsa and sauce, and substituted for salsa or enchilada sauce in most recipes. Just make sure the salsa verde you buy doesn't have peppers or other spices that might be triggers for you.

Makes 6 servings (2 enchiladas each).

- 4 chicken breasts, boneless and skinless (1 lb.)
- Chicken broth (enough to cover chicken—about 2–4 cups)
- 2/3 cup chopped green onions, white and part of green (if tolerated)
- 8 oz. grated reduced-fat Monterey Jack or cheddar cheese (or a mixture)

- 12 corn tortillas or high-fiber flour tortillas
- 1/4 cup milk or chicken broth
- 1 cup of bottled mild salsa verde (made with toma-tillos, onions, some peppers, salt, and cilantro)
- 1 cup fat-free or light sour cream

1. Add chicken breasts to a medium saucepan and add enough chicken broth to cover. Bring to a boil, then reduce heat to a simmer until cooked throughout (about 20 minutes). Let cool in chicken broth. Shred with hands and toss in a medium bowl with onion if tolerated, and the grated cheese.

2. Preheat oven to 375 degrees. Coat a 9 × 13-inch baking pan with canola cooking spray.

3. One by one, heat tortillas in a nonstick frying pan until softened. Lay about 1/3 cup of chicken mixture down the center of each tortilla. Add a tsp. of milk or chicken broth down the center, roll up, and place seamside down in the baking pan.

4. Cover the pan with foil and bake for 20 to 30 minutes.

5. Add salsa verde and sour cream to a mixing bowl and beat on low with mixer (or by hand) until combined. Spoon green sauce over the chicken enchiladas before serving, then pass any remaining sauce around the table.

Per serving (using flour tortillas): 470 calories, 35.5 g protein, 51 g carbohydrate, 13 g fat, 5 g saturated fat, 70 mg cholesterol, 3 g fiber (if corn is used), 715 mg sodium. Calories from fat: 25 percent.

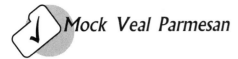

Mock Veal Parmesan

Makes 4 servings.

- 4 chicken breasts, boneless and skinless
- 1/2 cup egg substitute
- 1 cup Italian seasoned breadcrumbs (plain can also be used)
- 1/2 tsp. garlic powder (if tolerated)
- 1 tsp. Italian herb seasoning
- 1 tsp. parsley flakes
- 1 Tbs. canola oil
- 1 cup carrot sauce (see recipe below)
- 4 oz. part skim or reduced-fat grated mozzarella cheese

Serving suggestion: Serve each chicken breast over 3/4 cup cooked whole grain blend fettuccini noodles.

1. Preheat oven to 350 degrees.

2. Place a chicken breast between two sheets of waxed paper. Pound the side of the chicken breast that used to have the skin with a meat mallet until it's about 1/4-inch thick (or even better, ask your butcher to do it for you).

3. Pour egg substitute in a small shallow bowl. In another bowl, blend breadcrumbs, garlic powder (if tolerated), herb seasoning, and parsley. Dip each breast in egg substitute then coat well with breadcrumb mixture.

4. Spread canola oil evenly over the bottom of a 9 × 9-inch baking dish. Place chicken breasts in pan. Bake for 20 minutes. Spread at least 1/4 cup of carrot sauce over each breast. Then sprinkle mozzarella cheese over the tops and bake another 10 minutes or until chicken

is cooked throughout and cheese is melted. Serve over cooked noodles if desired.

Per serving: 416 calories, 42 g protein, 26 g carbohydrate, 15 g fat, 5.5 g saturated fat, 95 mg cholesterol, 2 g fiber, 1150 mg sodium. Calories from fat: 32 percent.

Carrot Sauce

Makes about 1 1/2 cups of sauce.

- 1 1/2 cups finely grated carrots
- 1/2 cup low-fat or whole milk
- 1 Tbs. butter or canola margarine
- 2 tsp. cornstarch
- 4 Tbs. low-fat or whole milk, divided use
- 3 Tbs. Parmesan cheese
- 1/2 tsp. oregano
- Pepper to taste

1. Puree grated carrots in blender or food processor with 1/2 cup milk. Melt butter on medium heat in large nonstick frying pan. Add carrot mixture and let bubble for a minute.

2. In small dish, blend 2 tsp. cornstarch with 2 Tbs. of the milk until smooth. Blend in remaining 2 Tbs. of the milk. Add to the carrot mixture, stir frequently, and let bubble a few minutes more. Reduce heat to simmer. Sprinkle cheese and spices on top, stir, and let simmer several minutes.

Light versions of 10 fatty foods

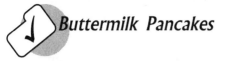

Buttermilk Pancakes

Starting the day off with a stack of rich pancakes, piled high with scoops of butter, all aside three greasy sausage links, can send your acid reflux into overdrive. Start the day off instead with a couple of light buttermilk pancakes, a nice drizzle of syrup, two lean links of sausage, and you'll be well on your way to a heartburn-free day.

Makes 5 servings (about 3 to 4 pancakes each).

- 1 cup cake flour (white flour can be substituted)
- 1 cup whole wheat flour
- 2 tsp. baking powder
- 1 tsp. baking soda
- 1/2 tsp. salt
- 2 Tbs. sugar
- 1 large egg
- 1/4 cup egg substitute (or 2 egg whites)
- 2 cups buttermilk (low-fat)
- 1 tsp. vanilla
- 2 Tbs. canola oil
- 1/4 cup reduced-calorie pancake syrup

Serving suggestion: Serve each stack of pancakes with a couple low-fat sausage links or patties (such as Jimmy Dean Lite Sausage with 50 percent less fat) and a small bowl of fresh fruit.

1. Combine flour, baking powder, baking soda, salt, and sugar in medium bowl and blend well with fork.
2. Beat eggs, buttermilk, and vanilla in mixing bowl on medium-low speed until smooth.

3. Add melted butter, pancake syrup, and dry ingredients to egg mixture in mixing bowl and beat on lowest speed, scraping with rubber spatula, just until blended. Do not over mix.

4. Let batter rest for 20 minutes. Spray griddle lightly with canola cooking spray. Preheat griddle until water skittles.

5. Pour 1/4 cup batter onto griddle. Cook over medium heat until bubbles form in pancake (30 to 60 seconds). Turn over with spatula and cook another 30 to 60 seconds or until golden brown

Per serving: 292 calories, 11 g protein, 46 g carbohydrate, 7.5 g fat, 1.3 g saturated fat, 46 mg cholesterol, 3.3 g fiber, 840 mg sodium. Calories from fat: 24 percent.

Light Denver Omelet

These omelets are great paired with the oil-free hash browns (recipe below).

Makes 2 fluffy omelets.

- 1 cup sliced fresh mushrooms
- 1 medium green pepper, chopped (as tolerated)
- 4 green onions, sliced diagonally (as tolerated)
- 1/4 tsp. dried basil, crushed
- 1/2 cup chicken broth
- 1/2 cup very lean ham cut into 1-inch long strips (about 2 oz.)
- 1/2 cup cherry tomatoes, halved
- 1/2 cup egg substitute
- 2 eggs, separated
- Canola cooking spray

1. Start heating a medium nonstick frying pan over medium heat and coat with canola cooking spray. Add sliced mushrooms, green pepper, green onions, and basil. Sauté about 20 seconds, then pour in 1/2 cup chicken broth and cook, stirring frequently, until tender. Stir in ham and cherry tomatoes and set mixture aside.

2. Blend egg substitute and egg yolks together in medium sized bowl and set aside. With mixer, beat egg whites until stiff. Carefully fold egg whites into egg-yolk mixture.

3. Generously coat a nonstick omelet pan or small frying pan with canola cooking spray and heat over medium heat. Spread half of egg mixture in pan. Heat until top looks firm (about two minutes). If your pan cooks hotter than normal, cook over low heat. Flip omelet over to lightly brown other side (about 1 minute). Fill with vegetable-ham filling, and fold as desired. Move to serving plate.

4. Repeat with remaining egg mixture.

Per serving: 188 calories, 22 g protein, 9 g carbohydrate, 7 g fat, 229 mg cholesterol, 2 g fiber, 690 mg sodium. Calories from fat: 34 percent.

Oil-free Hash Browns

Makes 2 servings.

- 2 cups frozen Southern Style Hash Browns (or 2 cups red potatoes, chopped in 1/3-inch cubes)
- 1 1/2 cups chicken broth (low sodium)
- 1/2 cup chopped onion (if tolerated)
- 1 or 2 cloves garlic (if tolerated)
- 1 Tbs. parsley flakes

Optional: 1/3 cup grated reduced-fat sharp cheddar cheese.

1. Heat broth, onion, garlic, parsley, and potatoes in medium saucepan until boiling.

2. Reduce heat to low and let simmer, uncovered, until water evaporates and potatoes are tender (about 15 minutes).

3. Add cheese if desired.

Per serving (with cheese): 255 calories, 10 g protein, 39.5 g carbohydrate, 6 g fat, 20 mg cholesterol, 220 mg sodium. Calories from fat: 22 percent.

Ham Skillet Breakfast

Makes one large serving.

- 1 medium boiling potato
- 1 egg
- 1/4 cup egg substitute
- 1 Tbs. low-fat milk
- 1 Tbs. finely chopped parsley (or 1 tsp. dried parsley flakes)
- 1/4 tsp. salt (optional)
- Freshly ground pepper (as tolerated)
- Canola cooking spray
- 1/4 cup finely chopped onions (as tolerated)
- 1/4 cup finely diced lean ham
- Water (if needed)

1. With a fork, pierce the potato three times. Place it on the microwave-safe dish and microwave on high until tender (about seven minutes). Set aside to cool.

2. With a plastic knife, peel the potato (if desired) and cut the potato into 1/4-inch slices; set aside.

3. In a medium bowl, beat the egg, egg substitute, milk, parsley, salt (if desired), and a few grindings of pepper with a fork until they are well blended.

4. Coat a nonstick skillet with canola cooking spray. Add the onion and ham and cook, stirring frequently with the spatula, over medium heat until onion is soft but not brown (about 5 minutes). Add a 1/4-cup of water if moisture is needed.

5. Add the potato slices to the onion/ham mixture and cook, turning occasionally with the spatula, over medium-low heat until they are light brown (about five minutes). Add 1/4-cup of water if moisture is needed.

6. Pour in the egg mixture. Tip the pan from side to side to spread the egg evenly. Reduce the heat to low and cook, without stirring, for 5 minutes. With the spatula, scoop up the underside of the mixture several times to prevent the eggs from sticking.

7. When the eggs are set, invert a serving plate over the skillet and, grasping the skillet and plate firmly together, quickly turn them over.

Per Serving: 383 calories, 23 g protein, 57 g carbohydrate, 6.8 g fat, 2 g saturated fat, 225 mg cholesterol, 5.5 g fiber, 590 mg sodium. Calories from fat: 16 percent.

Macaroni Salad for Purists

This is a no frills recipe for macaroni salad. But because of its simplicity, it is real easy to make and appeals to kids and discerning grown-ups alike.

Makes 8 side servings.

- 3 hard-boiled eggs
- 2 cups dry macaroni noodles (whole wheat or whole wheat blend)
- 3 green onions, white and part of green, finely chopped
- 2 tsp. parsley flakes, or 2 Tbs. fresh, finely chopped parsley
- 1/4 tsp. salt
- Freshly ground pepper to taste
- 2 Tbs. real or light mayonnaise
- 1/4 cup light or fat-free sour cream

1. Start boiling your eggs if you haven't done this already. Then boil the macaroni noodles following directions on box (boil about 8 to 10 minutes). Drain noodles well and rinse with cold water and let cool.

2. Place noodles in serving bowl along with green onions, parsley, salt, and pepper to taste. In small bowl, blend mayonnaise with sour cream; add mayonnaise mixture to the noodles in serving bowl.

3. Peel shells off eggs and remove two of the cooked yolks (discard other yolks). Chop remaining eggs and stir into macaroni mixture. Add more salt and pepper if needed to taste. Let sit in refrigerator overnight (if you've got time).

Per serving: 145 calories, 5.5 g protein, 21.5 g carbohydrate, 3.8 g fat, .7 g saturated fat, 28 mg cholesterol, 5 g fiber, 128 mg sodium. Calories from fat: 24 percent.

Spicy Steak Fries

Once you've tried these, you won't go back to deep-fried again. If you don't tolerate seasoning salt well, add salt and any herb blends that you like in its place.

Makes 6 servings.

- 4 medium to large russet (baking) potatoes
- 1 Tbs. canola oil
- Canola cooking spray
- 1/2 tsp. seasoning salt and add more to taste

1. Scrub the potatoes and cut them crosswise in half. Place cut-side down on a cutting board and use an apple cutter/corer to cut into wedges. If time permits, soak the potatoes in cold water for up to one hour to remove excess starch; drain and dry well.

2. Preheat oven to 425 degrees. Coat the bottom of a 9 × 13-inch baking pan or small cookie sheet with 1 Tbs. of canola oil.

3. Place the potato wedges in the pan. Spray the tops of the fries generously with canola cooking spray. Bake for about 20 minutes. Flip the fries over, sprinkle with salt, and bake for 10 minutes more, until lightly browned.

Per serving: 203 calories, 3.5 g protein, 41.5 g carbohydrate, 2.4 g fat, 0 g saturated fat, 0 mg cholesterol, 4 g fiber, 204 mg sodium. Calories from fat: 11 percent.

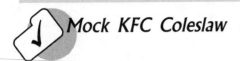

Mock KFC Coleslaw

Makes 8 side servings.

- 1/3 cup sugar
- 1/2 tsp. salt
- 1/8 tsp. freshly ground pepper (if tolerated)
- 1/4 cup low-fat milk (whole can be substituted)
- 2 Tbs. real or light mayonnaise
- 6 Tbs. fat-free or light sour cream
- 1/4 cup low-fat buttermilk
- 1 1/2 Tbs. white vinegar (seasoned rice vinegar can be substituted)
- 2 1/2 Tbs. lemon juice
- 8 cups finely chopped or shredded cabbage (about 1 medium head)
- 1 cup grated carrots

1. In a large mixing bowl, combine the sugar, salt, pepper, milk, mayonnaise, sour cream, buttermilk, vinegar, and lemon juice and beat on low speed until smooth.

2. Add cabbage, carrots, and toss to blend with dressing. Cover and refrigerate until served.

Per serving: 99 calories, 2.5 g protein, 17 g carbohydrate, 3 g fat, .5 g saturated fat, 3 mg cholesterol, 2 g fiber, 190 mg sodium. Calories from fat: 27 percent.

Southern Fried Chicken (oven fried, that is)

Fried chicken is one of America's all-time favorite fried foods. So, of course, I couldn't talk about lightening 10 fatty foods without including it. This is a nice, mildly spiced recipe. If you want to crank up the seasonings, add 1 tsp. of Creole or Cajun seasoning (if you tolerate this well).

Makes 4 servings.

- 4 chicken breasts, skinless (with bone or boneless as desired)
- 1 cup low-fat buttermilk
- 1–2 tsp. canola oil (for greasing bottom of baking sheet)
- 1 cup unbleached flour
- 1/2 tsp. fresh cracked black pepper
- 1/2 tsp. kosher salt (regular salt will work too)
- 1/4 tsp. cayenne pepper
- Cooking spray

1. Wash the chicken pieces and dry well with paper towels. Place the chicken in a gallon-size Ziploc bag and pour the buttermilk over the chicken. Seal the bag well and refrigerate for at least 30 minutes.

2. Preheat oven to 400 degrees. Add 1 to 2 tsp. of canola oil to cover bottom of a 9 × 9-inch baking dish.

3. Place the flour, pepper, salt, and cayenne pepper in another gallon-size Ziploc bag and shake to blend the ingredients.

4. Drain the chicken pieces briefly, then place one piece at a time in the bag filled with seasoned flour. Shake the bag vigorously to coat the chicken well; place chicken in prepared baking dish.

5. Coat the top of the chicken pieces with a generous coat of canola oil spray. Bake in center of oven for 20 to 25 minutes or until the chicken is nicely browned on the outside and cooked throughout on the inside.

Per serving (using 1 tsp. of canola oil to coat pan): 215 calories, 29.5 g protein, 13 g carbohydrate, 4 g fat, .6 g saturated fat, .5 g fiber, 69 mg cholesterol, 600 mg sodium. Calories from fat: 18 percent.

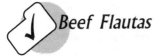

Beef Flautas

In Spanish, *flauta* means "flute." These meat-filled tortillas are rolled up like a flute and deep-fried until crispy. In this recipe we are oven frying the flautas until crispy, and using a lot less oil.

Makes 6 long flutes.

- 1 lb. extra-lean ground beef
- 1 medium onion, chopped (delete if not tolerated)
- 1 tsp. bottled minced garlic
- 1 1/2 tsp. chili powder (delete if not tolerated)
- 1 tsp. dry oregano leaves
- 1/2 tsp. paprika
- 1/4 tsp. ground cumin
- 1/4 tsp. pepper
- 2 tsp. Worcestershire sauce
- 1/2 cup mild chili sauce (or salsa verde or fat-free sour cream if not tolerated)
- 12 corn tortillas
- Canola cooking spray

Serving suggestion: guacamole (and mild salsa if tolerated well).

1. Preheat the oven to 400 degrees. In the skillet, place the ground beef, onion, and garlic. Brown the ground beef over medium-high heat, crumbling the meat into small pieces, using the spatula, as it cooks.

2. Add the chili powder, oregano, paprika, cumin, pepper, Worcestershire sauce, and chili sauce to the browned beef and stir.

3. Place six of the corn tortillas at a time into the damp kitchen towel and warm them in the microwave on medium for about two minutes. (If you don't have a microwave, you will need to heat one tortilla at a time in an ungreased frying pan over medium heat until flexible, about 15 seconds per side.)

4. For each flauta, spray both sides of two tortillas lightly with canola cooking spray. Lay the tortillas down so they overlap by 4 inches. Spoon 1/4-cup of filling down the middle of the paired tortillas and roll up tightly. Place on thick cookie sheet. Bake the flautas in the preheated oven until the tortillas are crisp (15 minutes).

Per serving (1 flauta): 248 calories, 15.5 g protein, 32.5 g carbohydrate, 6.5 g fat, 4 g fiber, 20 mg cholesterol, 280 mg sodium. Calories from fat: 24 percent.

Mini Corn Tamales

Traditionally, tamales are wrapped in soaked cornhusks and steamed. But to make this recipe quick and easy for you to make, the tamales are wrapped in squares of foil. Make a batch, then unwrap the cooled leftover tamales, and keep them in a Ziploc bag in the freezer. For a quick lunch or dinner, just take out as many tamales as you need from the freezer and warm them up in the microwave (about four minutes for two tamales).

Makes 24 mini tamales.

- 2 cups *masa harina* (corn tortilla flour)
- 1 1/4 cups chicken broth (double strength if possible)

- 1/2 tsp. salt (optional)
- 3 Tbs. canola oil
- 1/4 cup nonfat or light sour cream
- 2 cups finely shredded roasted or barbecued skinless chicken breast
- 2 1/4-oz. can sliced or chopped olives (optional)
- 1 medium onion, finely chopped (if tolerated)
- 1/2 cup bottled enchilada sauce, salsa verde, or low-fat gravy (if tolerated)
- Boiling water

Note: If tomato or tomatillo products are not tolerated well, use 1/2 cup of a gravy in place of the enchilada sauce or salsa.

1. Make 24 pieces of foil: Pull a strip of foil out of the box about 6 inches and carefully tear. Cut this in half to make two squares from the rectangle. Do this 11 more times to make 24 squares.

2. In a large mixing bowl, measure and combine the masa harina, chicken broth, salt (if desired), oil, and sour cream. With the electric mixer, beat briefly to make a thick paste. Spread 1 heaping tablespoon of the paste in the shape of a 3-inch square in the center of each piece of foil.

3. In another bowl, combine the chicken, olives, and onion. Add the enchilada sauce or salsa (or gravy) and with the large spoon, toss everything together. Spoon a heaping tablespoon of the chicken filling into the center of each masa square. Fold the foil edges together so the masa edges meet. Wrap the long end of the foil around each other and twist the ends.

4. Place a wire rack in a saucepan and pour in boiling water to a depth of 1 inch. The water should not

reach the tamales; if the rack is too low, rest it on two small cans. Stack the tamales on the rack, arranging them loosely so steam can circulate. Bring to a boil, cover, and adjust the heat to keep the water at a steady boil. Continue to cook, adding boiling water to maintain the water level, until the masa is nicely firm and does not stick to foil (test one from the center of the pan after one hour of steaming).

Per serving (2 mini tamales): 161 calories, 10 g protein, 17.5 g carbohydrate, 5.5 g fat, 2.5 g fiber, 20 mg cholesterol, 190 mg sodium. Calories from fat: 32 percent.

5 desserts that have nothing to do with chocolate and peppermint

Key Lime Bars

I'm a lemon bar and key lime pie lover from way back. So, it took me mere minutes to work up a lighter version of this key lime bar recipe. I love the idea of marrying the classic lemon bar recipe with a key lime pie. I was worried that I would be disappointed after this big buildup of taste expectation, but not to worry; these key lime bars are yummy. The shortbread cookie crust was tender and tasty and the lime topping was just the right amount of tart and tang.

Makes 12 large or 24 small bars.

- 3 Tbs. butter or canola margarine, softened
- 3 Tbs. light or fat-free cream cheese
- 1/2 cup granulated sugar
- 1 egg yolk
- 3/4 cup unbleached flour
- 2 Tbs. powdered sugar

- 1 egg
- 1/4 cup egg substitute
- 1 cup granulated sugar
- 2 Tbs. unbleached flour
- 1/3 cup key lime juice (regular lime juice may be substituted)
- 2 Tbs. powdered sugar (for sprinkling or sifting on top before serving)

1. Preheat oven to 350 degrees. Coat 8 × 8-inch baking dish with cooking spray..

2. In electric mixer, beat the butter, cream cheese, and 1/2 cup of sugar until light and fluffy. Beat in the egg yolk and gradually add the 3/4-cup flour. Spread into the prepared 8 × 8-inch pan. Sprinkle powdered sugar on top of the dough so the dough doesn't stick to the palm of your hands as you pat it down to make a crust in pan. Bake 15 minutes.

3. Meanwhile, in a mixing bowl (you can use the same one you used to make the crust), beat the egg and egg substitute slightly. Add in 1 cup of sugar and 2 Tbs. flour and beat on low speed until blended. Add the lime juice and beat on low until blended. Pour onto warm shortbread crust and bake for 15 minutes more.

4. Place on rack to cool. Before slicing and serving, sprinkle the top with 2 Tbs. or more of sifted powdered sugar.

Per large bar (if 12 bars per recipe): 180 calories, 2.6 g protein, 33 g carbohydrate, 4.5 g fat, 2.5 g saturated fat, 45 mg cholesterol, .3 g fiber, 55 mg sodium. Calories from fat: 22 percent.

Creamy Cherry Pie

This pie was a breeze to make. No pastry pie crust to blend and roll (you make a graham cracker crust). And the filling just calls for four ingredients, three of which are extremely convenient (sweetened condensed milk, a carton of sour cream, and a can of cherry pie filling). About the only thing you have to do is squeeze a couple of lemons. But if you buy bottled lemon juice, you don't even have to do that!

Makes 12 servings.

Crust:

- 1 Tbs. butter or canola margarine, melted
- 2 Tbs. fat-free or light sour cream
- 1 Tbs. lemon or orange liqueur (Grand Marnier or Caravella)
- 1 1/4-cup graham cracker crumbs

Filling:

- 14 oz. can fat-free sweetened condensed milk
- 1/4 cup lemon juice
- 1 cup of fat-free or light sour cream
- 21 oz. can of cherry pie filling

1. Preheat oven to 400 degrees. Coat the bottom and sides of a 9-inch deep-dish pie plate with canola cooking spray.

2. Combine butter, 2 Tbs. fat-free sour cream and lemon or orange liqueur in a food processor and pulse briefly just until blended. (If you don't have a food processor, blend the sour cream, liqueur, and butter together in a cup until smooth then drizzle it over the graham cracker crumbs in a medium bowl and stir well until completely blended.) Press mixture in

bottom and partway up the sides of a 9-inch pie plate and set aside.

3. Add sweetened condensed milk, lemon juice, and 1 cup of fat-free sour cream to mixing bowl and beat on low until smooth and creamy. Spread mixture over prepared crust.

4. Spoon cherry pie filling over cream mixture using small dinner spoons. Bake for 18 minutes or until filling appears to be nicely set. Let cool for about 30, minutes then refrigerate to cool completely. When ready, cut into 12 wedges.

Per serving: 239 calories, 5 g protein, 49 g carbohydrate, 2.3 g fat, 1 g saturated fat, 3 mg cholesterol, .7 g fiber, 140 mg sodium. Calories from fat: 9 percent.

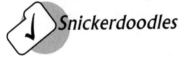

Snickerdoodles

I know chocolate chip cookies are the most popular cookie, but if you are avoiding chocolate—snickerdoodles have got to be a close second. They stay moist for days but I highly recommend you try them fresh from the oven.

Makes 3 dozen.

- 1/2 cup butter
- 1/4 cup light corn syrup
- 1/4 cup light cream cheese (in block)
- 1 1/4 cup white sugar (3/4 cup sugar and 1/2 cup Splenda can be used)
- 1 egg
- 2 egg whites
- 2 tsp. double strength vanilla extract (regular can be used)

- 1 1/2 cup unbleached white flour
- 1 1/4 cup whole wheat flour
- 2 tsp. cream of tartar
- 1 tsp. baking soda
- 1/4 tsp. salt
- 3 Tbs. white sugar
- 3 tsp. ground cinnamon

1. Preheat oven to 400 degrees. Coat a thick cookie sheet with canola cooking spray.

2. Cream together butter, corn syrup, cream cheese, and 1 1/4 cups sugar in mixer on medium speed. Add the egg, egg whites, and the vanilla and beat until blended.

3. Add the flour, cream of tartar, soda, and salt to mixing bowl. Beat on low speed to form a dough. Refrigerate for 2 hours or until firm enough to handle.

4. Add 3 tablespoons of sugar and cinnamon to small, shallow bowl and blend well.

5. Use a cookie scoop (1/8 level cup or heaping tbs.) to form cookie balls and roll each generously in the cinnamon sugar mixture. Place on cookie sheet, 2 inches apart. Bake about eight minutes or until set, but not too hard. Remove immediately from cookie sheet.

Per cookie: 99 calories, 1.5 g protein, 17 g carbohydrate, 2.9 g fat, 1.7 g saturated fat, 13 mg cholesterol, .3 g fiber, 90 mg sodium. Calories from fat: 26 percent.

Raspberry Coconut Bars

Raspberry bars—not to be confused with the more famous lemon bars. These bars have coconut and chopped pecans and are topped with a thin baked meringue type topping. I couldn't even tell the light rendition of these bars were light. I love this recipe!

Makes 24 bars.

- 6 Tbs. butter or canola margarine, softened
- 6 Tbs. light cream cheese
- 1 1/2 cups sugar (1 cup sugar and 1/2 cup Splenda can be used)
- 2 eggs, separated
- 3/4 cup white flour
- 3/4 cup whole wheat flour
- 3/4 cup raspberry preserves (low-sugar preserves will bring down the calories from sugar even farther)
- 1/2 cup shredded coconut
- 3/4 cup chopped pecans

1. Preheat oven to 350 degrees. Coat a 9 × 13-inch baking pan with canola cooking spray.

2. In electric mixer, beat the butter, cream cheese, and 1 cup of sugar until light and fluffy. Beat in egg yolks and gradually add the flour. Spread into prepared pan and bake for about 15 minutes. Cool slightly and spread with raspberry preserves; sprinkle with coconut.

3. Beat egg whites until stiff. Gradually beat in the remaining 1/2-cup sugar until soft peaks form. Gently fold in the pecans. Spread mixture over the raspberry preserve layer and bake again at 350 degrees for eight to 10 minutes or until top is lightly golden brown. Cool and cut into 24 bars.

Per serving: 170 calories, 2 g protein, 26.5 g carbohydrate, 6.5 g fat, 3 g saturated fat, 26 mg cholesterol, 2 g fiber, 56 mg sodium. Calories from fat: 35 percent.

Apple Crisp

You can make lots of variations with this recipe. For example, instead of apples, you can use 6 cups peach slices and 2 cups raspberries for a colorful, tasty crisp.

Makes 9 servings.

- 6–8 cups sliced apples, peeled or unpeeled depending on your preference
- 6 Tbs. whole wheat flour
- 6 Tbs. white flour
- 3/4 cup old-fashioned oats
- 3/4 cup packed dark brown sugar
- 1/2 tsp. salt
- 3/4 tsp. ground cinnamon
- 1/4 tsp. allspice
- 4 Tbs. butter or canola margarine, melted
- 1 tsp. vanilla
- 2 Tbs. buttermilk (regular milk can also be used)

1. Preheat oven to 375 degrees. Coat 9 × 9-inch baking dish with canola cooking spray. Place apple slices into prepared dish.

2. In medium bowl, blend dry ingredients. In 1 cup measure, blend butter, vanilla, and buttermilk together with fork. Drizzle butter mixture over the top of the dry ingredients and blend mixture with fork until the mixture is crumbly.

3. Sprinkle crumb mixture evenly over the fruit. Bake for 30 to 35 minutes or until apples are tender and top is lightly browned. Serve warm with light vanilla ice cream if desired.

Per serving: 206 calories, 2.5 g protein, 37.5 g carbohydrate, 6 g fat, 3.3 g saturated fat, 14 mg cholesterol, 4 g fiber, 14 mg cholesterol, 179 mg sodium. Calories from fat: 25 percent.

High-Fiber French Toast

This is one of those times when you want your bread to be sturdy so it can hold its shape when soaked with the egg mixture.

Makes about 4 servings (2 slices each)

- 4 large eggs (higher omega-3 if available)
- 1/2 cup egg substitute
- 1 1/2 cups fat-free half and half or low-fat milk
- 1 Tbs. pure vanilla extract
- 1 Tbs. liqueur of choice (grand marnier, amaretto, and so on)
- 1 Tbs. sugar
- 1/2 teaspoon ground cinnamon
- 1 pinch freshly grated nutmeg (or cinnamon if nutmeg bothers your stomach)
- 1 pinch of salt
- 8 large slices of whole grain or multigrain bread (any type you desire), cut 3/4-inch to 1-inch thick slices (day old works best)
- Canola cooking spray

1. Add eggs, egg substitute, fat-free half and half or low fat milk, vanilla, liqueur, sugar, cinnamon, nutmeg and salt to mixing bowl and beat until smooth and blended.

2. Start heating a large nonstick skillet over medium heat. Holding one of the slices with your left hand, submerge one of the bread slices in the egg mixture

and let it soak it up for about 10 seconds. Carefully lift the bread slice out (it will feel a lot heavier than it did going in) while you, using your right hand, generously spray an area (the size of the bread slice) on the hot skillet with canola cooking spray. Place the bread slice into the pan and repeat the steps with a couple more slices (until the skillet is full). Give the tops of all the slices a generous coating of cooking spray.

3. Panfry the slices until the bottom is golden brown (about two minutes) then flip them over to brown the other side (about two minutes more).

4. You will probably have enough egg mixture to make two more batches of French toast (about nine thick slices).

Per serving: 306 calories, 11 g protein, 50 g carbohydrate, 7.5 g fat, 2.8 g saturated fat, 3 g monounsaturated fat, 1.5 g polyunsaturated fat, 117 mg cholesterol, 5 g fiber, 358 mg sodium. Calories from fat: 22 percent.

Spinach and Mushroom Breakfast Bagel Sandwich

Makes 1 serving

- 3/4 cup sliced fresh mushrooms (crimini or regular)
- 1 whole grain or whole wheat bagel
- 6 Tbs. egg substitute (that is, Egg Beaters)
- 1/4 cup frozen chopped spinach, thawed and gently squeezed of extra water (or 1/2 cup fresh spinach leaves)
- Black pepper to taste
- 2 teaspoons freshly chopped (or frozen and thawed) chives

- 3 Tbs. shredded part-skim Jarlsberg or reduced-fat Swiss cheese

1. Add mushroom slices to a small nonstick frying pan coated with canola cooking spray and sauté until nicely brown (about three minutes). Meanwhile, slice bagel in half and place in the toaster or toaster oven.

2. Add egg substitute to 5-inch diameter microwave safe ramekin or custard cup coated with canola cooking spray. Stir in spinach (if using frozen chopped spinach) and microwave on high for one minute. Sprinkle black pepper to taste over the top and freshly chopped chives.

3. Assemble bagel by placing cheese and browned mushrooms over the toasted bagel bottom, and then top with the hot egg patty. If using fresh spinach, top the egg patty with the spinach leaves and tomato (if desired). Top with the other half of the toasted bagel. The Swiss cheese should melt nicely in the sandwich.

Per sandwich: 437 calories, 31 g protein, 66 g carbohydrate, 6.7 g fat, 3.7 g saturated fat, 1.5 g monounsaturated fat, 1.5 g polyunsaturated fat, 14 mg cholesterol, 12 g fiber, 890 mg sodium. Calories from fat: 14 percent.

Garlic and Herb (higher fiber) Pizza Crust

Makes 4 servings

- 1/2 cup + 3 Tbs. water, warm or room temperature
- 1 1/2 teaspoons molasses
- 4 tsp. extra-virgin olive oil
- 1 Tbs. minced garlic
- 1 Tbs. fresh, finely chopped basil (or 1 teaspoon dried)

- 1 Tbs. fresh, finely chopped oregano (or 1 teaspoon dried)
- 3/4 cup plus 2 tablespoons whole-wheat flour
- 1 cup white flour
- 1 tsp. salt
- 1 1/2 tsp. rapid rise or bread machine yeast

1. Add water, molasses, olive oil, garlic, basil, and oregano to bread machine pan (unless a different order is recommended by manufacturer). Add both types of flour to pan, and add the salt in one of the corners. Make a well in the center of the flour and pour in the yeast.

2. Select the dough cycle and press start.

3. When the dough cycle is complete, about 1 hour and 40 minutes, divide dough into four pieces. Press and stretch each piece out into a circle about 7 inches wide. Top with your desired sauce (pizza sauce or pesto) and toppings (cheese, veggies, and so on).

4. Bake the mini pizzas in a 400-degree oven until crust is golden brown, about 12 to 15 minutes.

Per serving (crust only): 250 calories, 7 g protein, 45 g carbohydrate, 5.5 g fat, 0.8 g saturated fat, 0 mg cholesterol, 4.5 g fiber, 538 mg sodium. Calories fat: 19%.

Yummy No Chocolate Brownies

This is a yummy dessert that has nothing to do with two potential heartburn offenders that are popular in the dessert department—chocolate and peppermint. Yes, I know, this recipe gives an option for white chocolate chips—but white chocolate really isn't chocolate, because it doesn't contain cocoa or cocoa butter.

Makes 12 servings

- 1/2 cup whole wheat flour
- 1/2 cup unbleached white flour
- 1/2 tsp. baking powder
- 1/8 tsp. baking soda
- 1/2 tsp. salt
- 1/3 cup no trans fat margarine with 8 grams of fat per Tbs.
- 1 cup packed dark brown sugar
- 1 large egg, high-omega-3 if available
- 1 Tbs. vanilla extract
- 1/2 cup white chocolate chips (optional)

1. Preheat oven to 350-degrees. Coat a 9-inch nonstick round or square cake pan with canola cooking spray.

2. Add flours, baking powder, baking soda, and salt to a 4-cup measure and whisk together well; set aside.

3. Melt the margarine in a small, nonstick saucepan over medium heat. Stir in brown sugar and continue to cook for about a minute. Remove from heat and let cool for a few minutes.

4. Add brown sugar mixture to large mixing bowl. Add in the egg and vanilla and beat on medium-low speed until well blended. On low speed, beat in the flour mixture, a little at a time, just until blended. Stir in the white chocolate chips if desired and pour into prepared pan.

5. Bake for 20 to 25 minutes or until brownies are done to your liking (don't overbake if you like them on the chewy side). Let cool about 10 minutes then cut into 12 squares.

Per serving: 115 calories, 2 g protein, 20 g carbohydrate, 3.5 g fat, .6 g saturated fat, 1.4 g monounsaturated fat, 1.3 g polyunsaturated fat, 21 mg cholesterol, 1 g fiber, 158 mg sodium. Calories from fat: 26 percent.

Slow Cooker Beef Stroganoff

Makes 4 servings.

- 1 1/2 pound eye of the round roast, cut into 2-inch long, 1-inch high and 1/4-inch thick strips
- 1 (10.75 ounce) can cream of mushroom soup with roasted garlic (condensed) or other cream of mushroom soup with around 2 grams of fat per soup serving (just check label)
- 3/4 cup chopped onion (delete if not tolerated well)
- 1 cup baby carrots (optional)
- 2 cups mushroom slices
- 1 Tbs. Worcestershire sauce
- 1/4 cup sherry or red wine (beef broth or water can be substituted)
- 1/4 cup light cream cheese
- 1/4 cup fat free or light sour cream
- Pepper to taste (salt to taste is optional)

1. In a slow cooker, combine the meat, consensed mushroom soup, onion, mushroom slices (if using raw), Worcestershire sauce and sherry.

2. Cook on the "low" setting for eight hours, or on "high" for about five hours. Stir in cream cheese and sour cream (and mushrooms if desired) just before serving. Add salt and pepper to taste.

3. Serve over hot, egg noodles, whole wheat pasta, white or brown

Per serving (not including noodles): 360 calories, 42 g protein, 18 g carbohydrate, 11.5 g fat, 5 g saturated fat, 101 mg cholesterol, 3 g fiber, 529 mg sodium. Calories from fat: 31 percent.

Chapter 7

Restaurant Rules

Dead man walking. Is that how you feel when you walk out of a restaurant after enjoying a rich, full meal, complete with several rounds of libations, late in the evening? It's hard to enjoy the moment of pure satisfaction after a wonderful meal when you know you are about to start paying (*big time*) for your dining indulgences—and I don't mean with your credit card. For many people, the heartburn starts to hit minutes after finishing their meal. Or, it could end up keeping you up all night.

Heartburn or no heartburn, many of us end up eating out many times a week, and restaurants definitely offer a few challenges. Once you know what your personal heartburn triggers and trouble foods are, eating out can be easier and a lot more comfortable, leaving two other important challenges:

- **Challenge #1:** most restaurant meals tend to be high in fat.

- **Challenge #2:** restaurant portions tend to be HUGE and if we clean our plate, so to speak, the large meal can increase pressure in the stomach, causing acidic stomach contents to splash back into the esophagus.

Dine smart

If you want to eat out in restaurants without suffering the consequences later (heartburn), avoid your triggers, avoid the higher fat menu items, and keep your meal size moderate by eating until you are "comfortable" and not "full" or "stuffed." Follow these five keys to heartburn-free dining.

Key 1: Select the right restaurant

Be sure you go to a restaurant that offers some acid reflux-friendly entrées or is at least willing to prepare an entrée per your special request. For example, if you have particular trouble with spices, a Thai restaurant may not be the best place for you. Or, if tomato, garlic, and onions get your goat, an Italian restaurant could be quite a challenge.

Key 2: Select the right menu item(s)

This sounds simple doesn't it? It's not. Here are just a few questions to ask your waiter. Remember, it never hurts to ask. The only thing you stand to lose is some extra fat and calories.

- Is this dish deep-fried?
- How is this dish prepared?
- Is there any butter or oil added?
- Is this made with mayonnaise?
- Is this made with cream?
- Can this be steamed, grilled, or broiled instead of fried or sautéed?
- Can I split an entrée with a friend rather than order a large meal on my own?
- Can I have the sauce/dressing on the side?
- Can this be cooked in wine or broth instead of butter or oil?

- Can this dish be broiled or baked instead of fried?

- Can you remove the skin from my chicken before it's prepared?

- Can I substitute a salad, baked potato, or steamed vegetables for the french fries?

- Can you make this dish without _____? (Insert whatever ingredient tends to aggravate your acid reflux, such as onion, garlic, or tomato.)

It goes without saying that you should order menu items that don't include the food ingredients that, without fail, help your heartburn along. If tomato products are a problem, don't go with the marinara or veal parmesan. If onions and spices spell t-r-o-u-b-l-e, then you might want to skip the 3-alarm chili. If you don't tolerate deep-fried foods well, order the grilled shrimp instead of the breaded or fried shrimp. You get the picture.

Key 3: Select the right amount of food

Remember sometimes it isn't as much "what" you eat, as much as "how much" you eat that can send you into heartburn overdrive. Granted, eating a smaller-sized meal is a real challenge when you are eating out—especially if you are in a "celebration mode." Because what do we do when we eat out? We eat foods we don't normally eat. We eat several side dishes or courses (soup, salad, and appetizers) before we even get to the entrée we've ordered. And we enjoy our food, usually not stopping until we are filled to the brim (marked only by needing to unfasten the top button on our pants). This will probably be the toughest key to follow, but the payoff is big.

Key 4: Eat early in the evening

For so many people with acid reflux, eating late in the evening is their biggest trigger with nighttime heartburn. Say your reservation is at 7 p.m. by the time you sit down, get a round of drinks, order your dinner, and finish up the meal, it could be 9 p.m. by the time you pay the check! Give yourself the requisite three to four hours before you lie down. So count back from when you want to go to bed and you may need to make that a 5:30 or 6 p.m. dinner reservation. Look on the bright side—you'll be able to get all those early bird prices on your favorite menu items.

Key 5: Chew on it a while, would you?

A little bit of gum chewing after a meal can go a long way with heartburn prevention. Keep a pack of gum in your purse or briefcase (or car as the case may be) and you might want to top off those restaurant meals with a big stick of gum—instead of a big cup of coffee or a plate of dessert. (For more on gum chewing being a heartburn helper, see page 48.)

5 rules for low-fat food in the "fast" lane

You've been driving for hours and now, quite possibly, you are in the middle of nowhere. Your stomach has been growling at you for miles, so you decide to get off at the next exit that has a fast food chain you recognize. That's one of the best things about fast food chains—reliability. You know what to expect whether it's a McDonald's in Nebraska or London.

Or, let's say you are running errands on your lunch hour, of which you only have 15 minutes left until you need to be back at the office. Where else can you pick up a meal in 10 minutes or less? If there is a drive-through window, you don't even have to leave your car if you don't want to. That's the other great thing about fast food—it really is fast! (The other thing about fast food is it's cheap—where else can you get lunch for $3 or less!)

Finding fast food isn't the problem when you have acid reflux—it's what to say when the person behind the window says, "Can I take your order?"

The biggest challenge for acid reflux sufferers eating at fast food chains is probably going to be avoiding high-fat foods. More than 12 years ago in my book on eating a low-fat diet without changing your lifestyle, I came up with "5 Rules for Feeding in the Fast Lane." And you now what, they still work.

Rule 1: Learn to limit total fat

Start off by ordering a sandwich or entrée with close to or less than 35 percent of its calories coming from fat. You are more likely to reach this mark if you:

- Go for the grilled chicken sandwiches instead of the fried.

- Avoid the "deluxe," "ultimate," or "double" burgers and sandwiches.

- Cut the cream and add your own salad dressing.

- Downsize instead of "super sizing" your order of french fries and other side dishes.

- Order the smallest hamburgers instead of the bigger kind—these have more bun per burger and tend to come with catsup and mustard instead of mayonnaise and "special sauce."

Rule 2: BYOP...bring your own produce

Look at any standard fast-food meal and think about the three calorie elements: fat, protein, and carbohydrate...and the major food categories (dairy, breads, fruits, vegetables, and so on) then ask yourself, "what's missing?" Sooner or later you'll arrive at the obvious; most fast food meals are sorely lacking in fruits and vegetables.

If you're lucky, some chains sell orange juice or let you make your own vegetable-packed salad. If not, you should plan to bring your own. "Bring vegetables and fruits with me?" you ask. I know this might take some getting used to. But it gets easier. I've found it's even contagious. Once you start doing this, you might find other coworkers and family members catching on too.

Fruits and vegetables (unless they are citrus fruits or tomatoes) generally don't cause trouble for people with acid reflux, and if your meal contains them, you are less likely to load up on the other high calorie, high fat, fast food meal items that could lead to trouble, so this point is worth practicing.

Practice #1

You just ordered the chicken breast sandwich from Wendy's along with a salad (using 2 tablespoons reduced calorie dressing). In this case, you are only missing your fruit. You can either bring a piece of fruit with you (banana, apple, peach, and so on) or buy a bottle of 100-percent juice or a piece of fruit at the market on the way, or bring it from home.

Practice #2

You've been sitting in traffic for hours. You are tired, frustrated, and starving. Just then you spot a Taco Bell in the distance. You decide to order the bean or combo burrito containing a bread/starch, some meat, or beans. But where's the fruit and vegetables? Looks like some carrot sticks and apple wedges are in order.

And remember to order your pizza with vegetables on top (skip the greasy pepperoni, salami, and sausage topping).

Rule 3: Dress your salad yourself

You may need to come equipped with some toppings. If the fast food chain you patronize doesn't offer a low calorie salad dressing, you still have these options:

- You can measure a couple of tablespoons of your own reduced calorie dressing from home into a small container and bring it with you.

- If you typically munch your fast food meal back at work, bring a bottle of your dressing to the office and keep it in the refrigerator.

Rule 4: Cut the cream (and opt for other condiments)

Many of these fast food sandwiches come with mayonnaise, and mayonnaise-laced sauces such as "special sauce" or tartar sauce. These sauces can send your sandwich into calorie and fat overload quicker than you can say, "hold the mayo." Just try squirting a little BBQ sauce, ketchup, or mustard on your sandwich instead. You can cut the fat grams in half just by having your Filet O' Fish without the tartar sauce.

Don't be afraid to order your sandwich without the mayo or special sauce. Or simply wipe it off the bun when you get it to your table.

What I like to do is tell them to add another condiment to the sandwich instead of the mayo. This seems to make them feel better—it's almost like they have to put something on the bun. So when I'm at the Wendy's drive through, I order the chicken breast filet sandwich with catsup, lettuce, and tomato instead of mayonnaise, lettuce, and tomato.

Rule #5: Once is enough!

When I was a kid we used to go to fast food when it was someone's birthday or something equally special. Today, people go on an almost daily basis. It's survival in this fast-paced world.

How much fast food is too much? It really depends on each individual. For my family, we try to go no more than once a week. This isn't necessarily because fast food is so "bad" for us (we can all make healthier choices when we go to get fast food), it's just that homemade food—eaten in a relaxed family environment—is so much "better."

If you put convenience first (maybe even cost) you might be driving through those Golden Arches almost every day. Not only does that encourage a total diet that is low in fruits, vegetables, fiber, and phytochemicals and rich in extra calories, fat, and sugar, but it makes fast food so standard, that it isn't special anymore.

What else should you know about fast food?

Besides the whole high-fat food thing, there are a few other things about fast food dining that can greatly challenge your desire to be heartburn-free.

- It's "fast food" after all, right? So guess what, we tend to eat our food—*fast*. Eating slowly will help the food go down in a relaxed manner. If we eat our meal slowly we may also avoid overeating. You have to give your stomach time to register to your brain that it's filling up. If you literally shovel it down in five minutes or less, you never give your tummy time to check in with your brain.

- How are you going to wet your whistle? Your beverage choices in fast food chains are limited to soda, coffee, and milk. The only other beverage I've seen offered is orange juice, and this high-acid drink may not be the best thing if you have acid reflux (it can bother some people). The calcium in milk can stimulate the stomach to release acid, so this may not work either. It is possible to order ice water—all you have to do is ask for it. I do it all the time.

- Everything about fast food is about *more, more, more.* Eating fast food is definitely going to test your desire to eat small-sized meals (and avoid eating *big*). I know this is cheating, but if I want a hamburger, I order the kid's meal hamburger. I get a nice, small hamburger (that automatically comes with ketchup and mustard instead of mayonnaise) and I get a few bites of fries (which is all I really want) and a drink. And even if I'm feeling like a chocolate shake, most of the chains will make you a kid-size shake instead of the drink. Again, this is just enough milkshake to satisfy me.

On the road is the worst!

When you have acid reflux and you are traveling for business or pleasure, this has got to be one of your most difficult times. All the acid reflux red flags are up and waving in your face.

You don't sleep well when you are traveling to begin with. Then your bed is flat and you don't have your special, extra fluffy pillow.

You are eating food you don't normally eat for starters. And you are eating out breakfast, lunch, and dinner, making it harder to follow the 10 Food Steps to Freedom.

Unless you want to eat alone, you have no choice but to follow the work crowd and eat those darn late dinners. When you are traveling on business, most of the dinner meetings are "late" dinner meetings. Then everyone hits the sack when they get back to the hotel room so they can be bright-eyed and bushy-tailed for the morning meetings.

Usually travel is stressful. Plane delays throw your eating and your comfort level off schedule. You wait in lines for everything. Then once you get there you are "on duty," answering questions about your project or products, meeting new clients, and so on. Any way you slice it, it's stressful.

So what can you do? Try your hardest to follow the 10 Food Steps to Freedom—especially now that you are traveling. And always carry some trusty medications with you, just in case.

More Americans are eating out than ever before!

While 7 percent said they buy at least one meal per day from a restaurant or store, 62 percent said they go out to eat weekly or more than once a week, according to a recent Allrecipes.com survey of more than 5,000 users. In the most recent government survey of food inakes, 57 percent of Americans ate at least one food away from home on any given day in 1994–1996. In 1977 to 1978, this number was 43 percent. (*Continuing Survey of Food Intakes by Individuals or CSFII*).

What do we eat then we go out?

For 32 percent of the people who took the 2006 Allrecipes.com survey, eating healthy, balanced meals is the biggest concern when eating out—and apparently some of us should be concerned.

The number-one choice for beverages is carbonated soft drinks, followed by coffee, then milk. Favorite foods for breakfasts eaten out include eggs, toast, pancakes, sausage, or bacon. The most popular vegetable items eaten away from home are lettuce salads, french fries, mashed potatoes, and coleslaw. And as far as main entrees go, pizza and pasta items such as spaghetti come up as popular items. (The 1994-1996 Continuing Survey of Food Intakes by Individuals or CSFII is the most recent government survey on this to date.)

Lower-fat and better-tolerated recipes for many of these favorite foods are featured in Chapter 6.

We generally eat more calories and fat when we eat out—simple as that. Studies show this again and again. Which makes sense because foods selected and eaten away from home have been reported as being higher in fat and cholesterol. But it isn't totally necessary to throw the baby away with the bath water. It's all about choices. What do you order when you eat out?

How much do we eat when we go out?

Using national survey data, researchers from the University of North Carolina at Chapel Hill discovered that portion sizes and calorie intake for specific food types have significantly increased over the years, with the greatest increases being for food eaten at fast food restaurants and Mexican food. (JAMA 2003, Volume 289 pages 450-453)

The *no-smoking* section please!

Request the no-smoking section in restaurants to ensure your comfort while dining. Remember that cigarette smoke increases the irritation to the esophagus as you breathe it in and out.

For your information

One-third of the people who ate out in 1994 and 1995 chose to eat at a fast food chain (which includes pizza parlors), according to a recent government survey. (Continuing Survey of Food Intakes by Individuals or CSFII.)

Index

A

acid of the stomach and foods that increase it, 69

acid reflux
- and asthma, 37-38
- and drugs, 22
- and relapse after healing the esophagus, 39
- and tests used to evaluate, 32
- and what's going on, 18
- and who has it, 17-18

acid reflux,
- complications of, 35-36
- cure for, 18-19
- the most serious complication of chronic, 36-37

183

About the Author

Elaine Magee is positively passionate about changing the way America eats—one recipe at a time! Her national column, *The Recipe Doctor*, appears in newspapers such as the *Atlanta Journal-Constitution, Democrat and Chronicle, Hartford Courant, Honolulu Advertiser*, and magazines such as *Today's Health & Wellness*. In the column—which she has been writing for the past decade—she performs recipe "makeovers," in which she is able to bring down the calories, fat, saturated fat, and sometimes sugar and sodium, while at the same time increasing fiber, phytochemicals, omega-3s, and monounsaturated fat. Elaine "doctors" real recipes while retaining the original good taste, and she keeps it easy. She believes that if there is a shortcut in the kitchen, you should take it!

Elaine is the author of more than 25 books on nutrition and healthy cooking, with her most recent book being *Food Synergy* (Rodale, March 2008). Elaine's medical nutrition series includes *Tell Me What to Eat If I Have Diabetes, Tell Me What to Eat If I Have Irritable Bowel Syndrome*, and *Tell Me What to Eat If I Have Acid Reflux*. Hundreds of thousands of these books have been sold, and they are now being distributed all throughout the world, including

China, Russia, Spain, Indonesia, and Arabic countries. New editions of these three books in the series will be released October–December 2008.

Elaine is a nutrition expert/writer for Webmd.com, SilverPlanet.com, and magazines across the country, and she appears frequently on radio, educational videos, and television shows. She has appeared on *Eye on the Bay* in San Francisco, the Fine Living Network, the *CBS Evening News*, *Mornings On 2* in San Francisco, and AM Northwest in Portland. She also conducted monthly healthy cooking segments for the Saturday morning news on NBC–San Francisco for two years. For two years before that, Elaine performed the "Light Cooking" segment for the KSBW-TV (NBC) midday news in Salinas, California. She was the writer and guest on a video with Teri Garr on multiple sclerosis and with Shekhar Challa, MD, on "The Heartburn Friendly Kitchen."

Elaine graduated as the Nutrition Science Department "Student of the Year" from San Jose State University with a bachelor of science in nutrition and a minor in chemistry. She also obtained her master's degree in public health nutrition from UC-Berkeley and is a registered dietitian. She was a nutrition instructor at Diablo Valley College for two years and the nutrition marketing specialist (California Department of Health) for the now national "5 a Day" health program for three years.

Other recent projects:

- Elaine is getting ready to launch her internet cooking show (stay tuned).
- Elaine was part of a satellite media tour in November 2007 on the topic of heartburn and the holidays.
- Elaine was the recipe developer for Pfizer pharmaceuticals, providing recipes to its website specific to three medical issues: high blood pressure, high blood cholesterol, and diabetes.